ALICE

ALICE

William E. Hermance, MD, FAAAAI
with Kim M. Hermance

Library of Congress Control Number: 2013906371
ISBN: Softcover   978-1-4836-2100-5
               Ebook   978-1-4771-7976-5

This book was printed in the United States of America.

Rev. date: 04/29/2013

To order additional copies of this book, contact:
Xlibris Corporation
1-888-795-4274
www.Xlibris.com
Orders@Xlibris.com
133110

Also by Dr. Hermance
"Tales from the Emergency Room"

The author wishes to thank Alice's grandmother (Grammy) whose cooperation was essential to the completion of this book and to whom it is dedicated with love and admiration.

Special thanks as well to Alice's parents for their inspiration, factual additions and critique of this story.

My appreciation also to William E. Powell, MD, FACOG (author of "From There to Here: Anatomy of a Divorce") for his efforts to improve the style and clarity of this story.

Table of Contents

PART II

Prologue

In a land far, far away, or perhaps, just next door, lived a girl called Alice. The experience of her birth left her so damaged that whether or not she would live became questionable. But, she did survive.

Here, then, is the true story of Alice's life from its problematical beginning to its tragic end. A story of the love of her family and friends. Really, in the end, it is a story of a happy life.

Though the names of people and places in the story have been changed, it is a cautionary tale for those responsible for the young lives of "special" children.

The range of emotions represented in this story is wide. Joy and happiness are paramount, as will be seen. Through it all however, there was never any anger, no thoughts of "why me?". Just an ordinary family trying to cope with extraordinary circumstances, emerging on the other side intact and with joy in the hearts of its members.

A Child of Mine (To All Parents)

I will lend you, for a little time, a child of mine, He said.
For you to love the while she lives, and mourn for, when she's dead.
It may be six or seven years, or twenty-two or three,
But will you 'till I call her back, take care of her for me?
She'll bring her charms to gladden you, and should her stay be brief
You'll have her lovely memories, as solace for your grief.
I cannot promise she will stay since all from earth return,
But there are lessons taught down here I want this child to learn.
I've looked the wide world over in search for teachers true
And from the throngs that crowd life's lanes, I have selected you.
Now will you give her all your love?
Nor think the labor vain
Nor hate me when I come
To take her home again?

I fancied that I heard them say,
"Dear Lord, Thy will be done!"
For all the joys Thy child shall bring,
The risk of grief we'll run.
We'll shelter her with tenderness,
We'll love her while we may,
And for the happiness we've known, forever grateful stay.
But, should the angels call for her,
Much sooner than we planned,
We'll brave the bitter grief that comes
And try to understand.

Adapted from: Edgar A. Guest
(Dicksons)

Part I

"I will instruct you and show you the way you should walk, give you counsel and watch over you."

Psalm 32:8

Chapter 1

Alice is Born

Robert and Millie Anderson were spending a few days at the home of friends on Cape Cod. It was a beautiful day in the fall, 1990, and another couple from Houston, Texas, was with them. Dr. and Mrs. Howell, Will and Jean, had been friends of the Andersons since college and medical school where Will and Robert were classmates. Dr. Howell was a very well-known obstetrician in Houston, Texas.

In the middle of the day, the Andersons received a call from their second oldest son, Gregory and daughter-in-law, Carol. Carol was pregnant for the first time, about three months along. She was having some spotting and had been to see her doctor. Apparently, there was nothing to worry about, but Carol was concerned.

Dr. Howell immediately listened to her story over the phone, agreed with her doctor and gave her encouragement based on his extensive experience with pregnant patients. No one heard any more about any problems. Carol's pregnancy proceeded normally thereafter.

Gregory and Carol, both known for their attention to detail, had done their research and had chosen a well-known and highly regarded, Board Certified OB-GYN physician, Dr. Jon C. Johnston. He was affiliated with the well-known Westside Hospital for Children.

Millie and Robert grew more excited as Carol's due date in early May drew closer. They were already the proud grandparents of Meghan Elizabeth Anderson, born to their oldest son, Robert, Jr. and his wife, Marie, in Texas. They remembered the joy surrounding her birth and the anticipation of their trip to Texas to meet her.

How different their experience of Alice's birth was going to be!

Usually, when the telephone on Robert's bedside table rang in the middle of the night, it would be a patient calling. But, on this night in early May 1991, it was his son Greg calling from the hospital. Clearly upset, he told his parents that his baby, a girl, had arrived. Instead of the happy son Millie and Robert were used to, Greg, who was always so supportive of others, was clearly in great distress and trying to hold back his tears, not very successfully. His mother and father tried to comfort him when he said, "Something is wrong with the baby." No one knew then what the problem was and so his parents could only try to reassure him. This is difficult to do in any meaningful way when there are virtually no facts available. Robert suggested that, just in case, Greg keep a complete diary of all events, noting especially the timing and sequence of these events, starting from the onset of Carol's labor. Carol eventually did the same, recalling as much of her experience as she could. This later caused one of the malpractice lawyers eventually involved to ask how it was that Greg knew the timeline of events so clearly. He noted that his father had suggested he keep a log.

Greg would call back.

The Andersons were devastated. Robert prayed the rosary right then that the baby would be all right.

What follows is the story of a neglected delivery.

Carol began her labor at about 2:00 am when her water broke. She was in her ninth month, at full term. She was asleep at the time. Her obstetrician was informed and she went to the hospital as instructed. At some point in the labor room it became clear that there was fetal distress. Fetal monitoring was ordered. Unfortunately, the labor rooms were all filled that night and there were not enough monitors to go around. One was eventually found for Carol, but this monitor was not functioning correctly, not to say that it was broken.

The obstetric's house staff was in communication with Carol's doctor. He suggested that her labor should continue, with monitoring. He did not immediately come to the hospital; no mention was made of a cesarean section.

Robert never saw the obstetrician, but he learned later that, at delivery, Carol's white blood cell count was 22,000 and the baby's count was high as well. Septicemia (blood-borne infection), then, was part of Alice's problem at birth. There had also been difficulty with the birth process, Carol's birth canal being somewhat narrower than would provide for an easy birth. It was clear that Alice's head was misshapen on the left side. It was later learned that a good deal of her brain was severely damaged. Finally, the fetal monitoring seemed to indicate that she had undergone a degree of oxygen deprivation. The monitor recordings would later play a significant role in the legal proceedings surrounding Alice's delivery.

So, here were several reasons why all was not well with the Anderson's grandbaby.

Carol was in labor for 22 hours including 18 hours after her water broke. This is an extraordinarily long time for labor to be left to continue, almost certain to result in perinatal infection probably of both mother and child. (Even many years ago all these problems could easily have been avoided in a normal, full-term pregnancy.)

Alice's grandmother, Millie Anderson (Grammy), made immediate arrangements to fly to The City. At the airport she was met by Alice's father. It was about 4 pm and they went directly to West Side Medical Center. First, they went to see Carol who was not doing well at that point and then to the neonatal unit. Outside the neonatal intensive care unit, Grammy came upon Alice's obstetrician. His comment, without any apparent evidence of concern for Millie's feeling was, "The mother is doing OK, the baby isn't." And with that he walked away. Grammy was furious following this encounter and one can only contemplate what might have happened to the doctor had he not left immediately.

As far as Carol knew, Alice's initial problem was seizures. Greg and Carol went down to the pediatric ICU to see Alice after an awful night of worrying—Carol in the hospital and Greg at home. It was one of the worst nights in Carol's life because she was hurting after an episiotomy. She prayed all night for God to just let her baby live. Later she told a Bible study class she was leading to "be careful of what you pray for: God answered my prayers, but, in retrospect, I should have prayed for Alice to be healthy!" In the end, Carol and Greg went to the neonatology unit to see Alice and left feeling relieved because, they were told, she was doing well.

Shortly thereafter, Alice started having seizures.

After Alice was born, her parents spent the first several days worried if she would even live. After many tests and after it became apparent Alice would make it, the question became what quality of life she would eventually have. Because of the initial seizures and other issues including an infection, Alice was on a lot of medication. At one point Carol remembers worrying about whether the baby even had the ability to suck on a nipple. So the Andersons waited as the medications were eliminated or the doses were lowered to see what abilities Alice still had, including a sucking reflex. They were called into a meeting sometime during the first week with the team caring for Alice after a developmental pediatrician examined Alice and looked at her brief but complicated medical history.

It was at that meeting the Andersons were first told that Alice probably would have cerebral palsy in the moderate to severe range and that she most likely would have developmental delays due to the loss of oxygen and other issues surrounding her birth. The doctors needed to see how she responded as the medications decreased and there were no certainties with regard to her prognosis or diagnoses. Some children did very well and had minimal problems and some did less well. Alice would require follow-up with the Rehabilitation Center initially so the staff could see how she was developing and, if necessary, early intervention services could be arranged. Already, they were encouraging the Andersons to bring toys in that had music or other toys such as black and white ones to stimulate Alice's brain. It was the start of a journey where every activity or interaction with Alice had a higher purpose. Play was almost always therapy.

The intensive care unit where Alice was being cared for was large, brightly lit, and filled with accommodations for many babies suffering various levels of distress. The area was filled with the noise of various machines and the nursing staff was in constant motion. One could barely see Alice for all the wires and machinery surrounding her.

After a while, Alice was moved from the "critical" area of the neonatal intensive care unit to another room that was lower in medical intensity. The nurses who were assigned to her care stayed with her. The nurses were the Anderson's lifeline—they were supportive, helpful and caring to Alice as well to Greg and Carol. They tried to provide them with experiences that were as normal as possible, such as giving Alice a bath or rocking her to sleep. Of course, it was hard to visualize rocking a baby to sleep who is attached to monitors with wires and IV's as a normal experience, but they tried. Carol remembered arriving one day early on, to find one of the nurses feeding Alice with a bottle. She was sucking, which was great news. The nurses seemed to have little techniques that helped these babies learn how to suck. For a while, Carol was pumping breast milk and bringing in the milk to the nursery so Alice could be fed her mother's milk while in the hospital. Carol tried to get Alice to breast feed when she first came home, but she could not seem to learn it now that she had learned how to suck on a bottle. It was disappointing, but for a while Carol continued to pump breast milk and then give it to the baby in a bottle which made feeding sessions twice as long. The helpful part though was that Greg could at least feed her in the evening after work or at night so that each parent could string together several hours of sleep.

Each of the nurses seemed to be personally involved with the babies and their families. They took great pride in saving the smallest of the preemies, and in trying to help the damaged babies. During her initial visit, the nurses were also concerned for Grammy's well-being. Millie remembers one of the nurses taking the time to tell her that she felt badly for grandparents in Millie's situation since they were concerned for the baby, their own children and under great emotional stress themselves.

After arriving at the hospital, the new father and Grandmother Millie revisited Carol and then went out for supper. Then, it was back to the hospital and finally on to Greg and Carol's house where Grammy remembers seeing a bottle of champagne wrapped in foil for a planned toast to the new baby. Today, she is not sure if it ever was opened.

As soon as possible, Robert drove to the hospital. It was a very long trip. Ordinarily, Millie would have been with him, so the trip was lonely, and given the circumstances, an unhappy one. Once there, it was difficult to see what this 6 lb. 2 oz. baby even looked like with so much equipment attached to her little body.

When Robert arrived, he was treated with the utmost respect as a physician. The staff should not have been concerned about his reaction to their efforts since they seemed to have everything under excellent control. Robert, a specialist in clinical allergy and immunology, a vastly different field of medicine of course, was mostly out of his element in this busy pediatric intensive care unit.

How far advanced things had become in this modern age was the fact that there actually were people who could be called upon to teach newborns to suck! Robert was flabbergasted. Alice might have become a candidate for this intervention, but her sucking reflex eventually proved to be normal. Her problem then and afterwards was learning to swallow.

After Henry and Helga MacDonald, Carol's parents, the "other" grandparents, had left for their home near East Vale, and after Robert had had a chance to see what the situation was with Alice, Greg, Carol, Millie and Robert found themselves alone in the house on Swanson Avenue in Maneta. They were trying to sort out just what Alice's condition really was when her mother, Carol, asked Robert a question he had been mulling over. What should be done if Alice never was able to be fed normally? Carol was asking from a medical viewpoint, he guessed. And so he said that, if it were up to him, the advice would be to not start feeding her parenterally (nutrition delivered bypassing the gastrointestinal tract). The implication of this became clear all too quickly. Carol, very smart, a strong, somewhat feisty young woman, perhaps feeling a dent in her emotional armor, went into the kitchen to try to get a handle on her sorrow—exactly as her husband and in-laws were trying to do. It isn't possible to put into words the sadness Robert felt making this suggestion. When Alice was weaned off of the medications she was given for the seizures, her sucking reflex kicked in so that she was able to take nourishment by mouth.

But, it wasn't easy. Despite Carol's efforts to have Alice fed her milk from breast pumping, it soon became obvious that Alice's swallowing mechanism was so uncoordinated that it was impossible for her to be fed liquids without having her aspirate (inhale) them—a very dangerous problem in anyone, especially an infant or small child. Alice had a swallowing study done when she was about a year old, because she was losing so much of the liquids she was drinking and because she was gagging on the baby food her parents were trying to feed her. Greg and Carol worried about Alice's hydration. Carol kept track in her head every day for Alice's whole life how many wet diapers they had changed so if she didn't urinate sufficiently, Carol would push liquids or pudding or ice cream. Also, from then on and for all of Alice's life, her liquids had to be thickened. Thankfully, a satisfactory thickening agent was available and so Alice was always satisfactorily hydrated.

After approximately 3 weeks, her parents took Alice home from the hospital. They were told to treat her like any other child and were given a follow-up appointment at the Rehabilitation Center in a few weeks to see how she was responding developmentally. At home, Alice was a very fussy child but, since she was their first, Carol and Greg didn't really have anything with which to compare the experience. Perhaps it was partly a lack of experience at handling babies but still, she was very much a challenge. First, Alice could not seem to relax enough to sleep for any length of time even at night. She took power naps of only 20 to 30 minutes if she was sleeping in her swing. She seemed to startle herself awake. At night, she might sleep longer, but again, she often would seem to startle herself awake or not be able to get comfortable. Greg or Carol would go in and switch her position for her. From one side to the other and arrange her legs. When she was older, she would often go right back to sleep assuming she wasn't ill with a cold, but as a baby she would often be awake at that point and it was very hard work to try to get her back to sleep. While this is true of most babies for a short time, the Andersons dealt with this for many years. Greg and Carol would alternate whose turn it was to go and re-position Alice so one of them could sleep a few hours. But they spent all of Alice's life sleep deprived. As a passenger in the car, Carol often would fall asleep within minutes. During her first summer, if Alice fell asleep, no matter where, no one moved or touched her. So her baby book has funny pictures of her cat-napping on couches or chairs, but very few pictures of her actually sleeping in her crib! Every once in a while, though, Alice would sleep 6 or 7 hours straight at the same time her parents were sleeping. It was a gift!

Soon, at the rehab center, when Alice was about 3 to 4 months of age her parents were told that she was not hitting developmental milestones at an appropriate time. They were advised to research and find an early intervention program that would work for them, and they were given a list of programs. There followed phone calls and appointments to check out various programs. They ended up choosing a program at the Center that would involve a teacher visiting their home 3 times a week for an hour and a bi-weekly visit to the center for a therapy clinic where a parent and Alice went to the therapy room and spent 20 to 30 minutes with an occupational therapist, physical therapist and speech therapist rotating through with other infants and their parents. The idea was that, as parents, the Andersons would take the techniques the teacher and therapists showed them and continue these "tricks" at home so as to encourage Alice to do basic developmental tasks such as rolling over, sitting up, or grasping an object.

At first, they tried to have daily therapy time at home, but found that did not work so well. It was easier just to work the various tasks into daily interactions with Alice. For example, Alice had a very strong reflex which resulted in one arm being bent at the elbow with a fisted hand by her ear. Her other arm would be locked straight out by her side. With her arms in these positions, she was not able to turn her head past the midline or the center of her body toward the side with the hand by her ear.

Brightly colored pictures and a musical wind-up toy were placed on the side of her changing table so she would try to turn her head to look at the pictures or listen to the music. Eventually her parents had to switch the side they changed Alice's diaper on or gave her a bath; learning to do it "backwards" so that, in order to look at them, Alice had to turn her head in the direction she was having trouble with. In another example, Alice's arms were very stiff and often straight by her sides with her hands fisted. She tried to bat at things or reach for things as if she was doing a straight arm front raise, fisted with her elbows locked. The whole time while feeding

Alice, time was spent playing with her hands, trying to peel open her hands by opening her hand finger by finger and then trying to bend her elbow.

One of the first things taught at the Program was passive stretching and range of motion exercises. Because of Carol's background as a student athletic trainer in college, she knew how important maintaining Alice's range of motion would be. The problem was that all of the stretches took a lot of time and initially Alice hated to do them. Possibly she felt pain doing them or just got bored doing them or both, but she would scream and cry at what seemed the top of her lungs. As if she was being tortured! Eventually, movements like bringing her arm over her head with her fingers and hand opened or bringing her leg up toward the ceiling then pointing and flexing her ankle and circling it as if it was the stretching done at the end of an aerobics class, were combined. Stretches were done as soon as she woke up—on the changing table, when she was in a crib and later in her bed. Barney songs, nursery rhymes, even songs from commercials were sung to help her relax and not cry while having her stretching exercises. Alice was stretched every morning for her whole life. She maintained a very good range of motion with the exception of her hamstrings and hip flexors in later years when she sat in her wheel chair so much. A level of flexibility was maintained so that surgical intervention was never needed. Other things were added so as to maintain leg flexibility such as AFO's (foot orthotics) to keep her ankle flexion present with lengthened calf muscles, a standing regimen, assisted swimming and even letting her lie on her back listening to music on the floor so she could stretch out her hips as best she could. But when one sits in a wheelchair for most of the day—it is hard to counteract the shortening of muscles with a twenty minute daily stretching session.

The teacher who came to the home to work with Alice was named Sue Fromme and was wonderful. She would arrive with several toys or tactile stimulation activities to help Alice learn cognitively as well as support the goals of her various therapies. Alice's teacher became a friend and Carol thought they helped each other to some degree. She taught Carol how to be a proactive advocate for Alice—skills that she used to keep Alice's goals moving forward her whole life. In a way, many of Alice's goals were the same her whole life. First, starting out trying to get her to reach out and grasp an object, progressing to reaching out and pushing a switch that would operate a toy. As a preteen, Alice was taught to reach out and push a button or switch so she could use her augmented communication device to choose an activity or tell others what she wanted to eat. What most kids could master fairly quickly, took Alice years of practice to perfect. But even though her progress was slow, she always did make progress. Sue also knew that all the learning and therapy had to be fun; knowing she needed many ideas to keep the sessions interesting and to keep the short attention span of a baby focused. Alice, for the most part, enjoyed her teaching sessions.

In the therapy clinic especially, physical therapy was another story. The therapists meant well, but they seemed to expect Alice to do the same task or activity over and over so that she would quickly become bored and start "screaming". Yes, screaming! Alice responded most negatively to physical therapy. It was almost as if she took an immediate dislike to the therapist. When she arrived at her station, Alice would start screaming. Alice and the therapist would literally seem to battle it out with the therapist insisting on doing something and Alice's resisting, becoming even more spastic than she usually was and roaring at the top of her lungs. With the other therapies, Carol could intervene a bit and get Alice to try for a while, but nothing she tried helped with physical therapy. Carol would often leave the therapy clinic and get in her car only to start crying because it was so upsetting. Over the years, the Andersons realized that Alice actually was a good judge of a person—she seemed to sense if a person was comfortable and at ease with her or themselves. There were other people she seemed to dislike and often, in the end, Carol would realize that Alice was a better judge of character than most people. So, Carol wonders to this day what Alice sensed about the physical therapist that Carol could never see. When eventually another therapist appeared, Alice reacted in a better fashion. So, it wasn't PT—it actually was the specific therapist.

Alice was very stubborn and she often did react strongly to new situations or things she did not want to do. Carol often told herself that it was Alice's stubbornness that saved her life, but when she would cry the minute her mother walked away from a table at a restaurant, it was very hard to be patient. She had become quite the Mommy's girl and she would have separation anxiety that involved major screaming that literally did not stop. They told any babysitters they had that Alice probably would scream the whole time, but to do their best. Most sitters were honest. Yes, she cried the whole time and she cried herself to sleep they would say, they tried to comfort her as best they could. They were paid generously so they would be willing to come back. One sitter though would always report she had no trouble. Alice was fine. Carol thought this sitter just had the special touch. She was a very experienced sitter even though she was a teenager. Until Carol and Greg came home shortly after leaving one time because they had forgotten something, to discover their daughter screaming in her crib with the babysitter watching TV. Apparently that was her solution, put her in the crib immediately and ignore her until she fell asleep. The Andersons learned to always make unannounced visits to the babysitters.

Developmentally, Alice did achieve a few milestones especially being able to smile and laugh. In November, when Alice was 6 months old her Dad was able to coax her first smile while playing with a stuffed pig which would make squeal noises. Once she figured out how to smile it wasn't very long before she learned to laugh. Again, her Dad was on a mission to change those smiles into chuckles. Her great big smile and a laugh that almost seemed to start at her toes would make friends and other adults laugh right along with her over her whole life. Her cerebral palsy made her muscle tone extremely high which meant she could use the tone to hold her head up or sit up with her stiff arms in front of her to help her balance. It wasn't the "normal" way to sit, but Alice learned to use her spasticity in some ways to her advantage. She hated to lie on her stomach as it was very hard for her to move her arms underneath herself to pick up her head, but she figured out how to roll over from her stomach to her back by arching as long as her arms were positioned for her. She never did learn to roll from her back to her stomach without assistance. On her back, she would move, rock and kick her way around in a circle like a clock but never could roll. She learned how to reach out for something, but never could actually grasp an object unless it was put in her hand. So, developmental steps were done with assistance. She learned about rolling with help. Play, such as feeding her baby doll, was accomplished with hand over hand assistance. It was challenging day to day because Carol would have to divide her time between helping Alice play and still try to get household chores done. Toys were purchased for the purpose of achieving some developmental milestone, not necessarily for the sheer pleasure of play. Alice's grandmothers were often tasked with looking out for a particular item or toy that would help Alice out. Greg's Mom was able to make a number of items to assist Alice. The most famous was the "hippo roll" so named because it was a rolled up pillow covered in fabric printed with pink and purple hippopotamuses.

During the first 14 weeks of Alice's life, Carol was at first on medical leave and then on unpaid family leave. Once the baby was home, life settled down, but in retrospect, Carol thinks she may have had a bout of depression or the post-baby blues which would not be unusual in a normal situation, but after the experience she had gone through, she had quite a challenge. At the time, neither she nor Greg appreciated Carol's depression, even though she would get nothing done during the day. Greg was coming home from work for lunch to find Carol in her PJ's still sitting watching TV. After taking care of Alice, Carol found it hard to do much else. She would take a shower when Greg got home and try to perk herself up enough to get dressed and accomplish something. Eventually, she started to come out of the place she was in, and she remembers consciously realizing she had to shut the TV off. Keeping the TV off helped her take steps to move in the morning. It was at that time that Carol adopted a policy that has served her well through many life challenges: she would try to get one thing, project or job accomplished each day even if it was something small like cleaning the bathroom. At least that way she could look back on the day and feel she had accomplished something positive. In September after Alice was born, Carol tried to go back to work full time. One of her co-workers had a sister whose daughter was born around the same time as Alice. Ashley had been born prematurely and while at higher risk for developmental delays, was progressing normally. Her mother wanted to continue to stay home with her and was looking for another infant to take care of for extra money. It seemed like the perfect situation because she also was trying to make sure the environment was supportive of strong developmental growth. So Carol changed her hours at work, starting at 7 a.m. so she could pick up Alice right after she got out of work at 3:30 p.m. Greg would get Alice up and drop her off at the sitter's which was on his way to work in the morning. This was a challenge for Carol. She is not a morning person, so trying to get to work at 7 am was stressful and she did not see Alice often in the morning. When she picked up Alice she usually had to take her immediately to therapy or get her home in time for the teacher to come. She and Greg were not sleeping at night more than 2 or 3 hours at a time because their daughter was such a challenging sleeper. The babysitting arrangement worked out extremely well as the sitter took great care of Alice, but still, they were stressed and sleep deprived. In addition there were many doctors' appointments to take Alice to, such as her pediatrician, the developmental doctor, and the eye doctor (Alice very obviously had a "lazy" eye) to name a few.

By Thanksgiving, Greg and Carol were arguing with each other quite a lot. Soon after, they realized that if the marriage was to survive and if they were going to concentrate on giving Alice the best they could, something had to change. Carol tried to propose working part time at her place of employment, but this was rejected. At the same time, Greg started a new, better paying job with his office located downtown in The City. So in January, Carol gave two weeks' notice and they decided to try to make it on one income. It was extremely tight budget-wise and they did run up too much debt (which eventually would get paid off when the law suit for the issues that occurred with Alice at her birth) was settled, but it was one of the smartest decisions they made. It took much of the day to day stress away, and Greg and Carol could concentrate on the marriage and being strong for their daughter. As a stay-at-home Mom, it meant Alice's therapy and teacher visits could be during the day when she was at her best. Carol joined a play group that gave her some socialization and helped Alice by allowing for her interaction with other kids. There was also a weekly program at church for Moms to socialize and do some bible study, which was helpful. The friends Carol made through church became a great support system for both Greg and her. Alice and her mother developed a routine for the day. When she would fall asleep for her 30 minute power nap, Carol would try to get some housework done. Carol says now, looking back, it was amazing at how fast she could clean a room in the house! Initially they had two cars but sometime in that first year, they moved to just one car when the lease on Greg's car was up. Carol used the only car since she needed to get Alice to her various therapies and appointments while Greg walked two blocks and caught the bus downtown.

One of the things Greg and Carol got right was the notion that they had to take care of themselves as much as possible so they could be good parents. Carol knew that she needed to have time for herself, to refill and reset her emotional and stress levels to be the best mom and wife she could be. Greg was really great about watching Alice for an hour while she went to a nighttime aerobics class twice weekly. She also tried to go for a run a couple of times a week. Her aerobics class or a run was a great mental reprieve from the stress of working while she was still employed and even when being a stay-at-home mom. They also purchased a Baby Jogger which they used as soon as Alice was big enough to fit into it. That way Carol could go for a run and take Alice along. Greg had gotten used to getting up in the morning early on to go for a run and he continued to get up at 5 AM to do his workout. Alice eventually adjusted to life in the baby jogger and ran in several 5K road races with her dad pushing her. The baby jogger came in handy for many other community outings over the years and the family purchased a special-order larger jogger for older kids with disabilities when Alice outgrew the initial one. They used the jogger at the beach, at parks, even going to cut down their Christmas trees over the years. Alice really enjoyed trips in the jogger that were bumpy—it made her laugh.

When one has a child with a disability, initially it is hard to watch other kids about the same age without feeling jealousy or anger as to why all of this had to happen to one's family and child. In retrospect, Carol says one actually goes thru a grieving process, mourning the child one thought one might have and dreamed about and then, slowly, coming to an acceptance of the new child. It is not an easy or smooth process. Greg and Carol remember one book in particular they read that first year that helped them come to terms with their new reality: "When Bad Things Happen to Good People" by Rabbi Harold S. Kushner. And while one does eventually, intellectually, begin to make sense of things, emotions are often harder. There are still the emotions; one just learns to respond to them intellectually.

The birth of their second child really helped them to heal. Carol got pregnant shortly after Alice's first birthday. She and Greg were so very excited, but at the same time very anxious that this second child would be healthy and normal. Alice was still going to the therapy clinics with her teacher coming to the house. Carol remembers how tired she was throughout her pregnancy because Alice was such a poor sleeper. The teacher would come to the house and Carol would attempt to stay awake and pay attention, but pretty quickly would fall asleep on the floor while Sue would be playing out her lesson plan with Alice.

Chapter 2

Medical Malpractice Lawsuit

Dr. Anderson didn't know just when the idea of a medical malpractice lawsuit arose in Alice's parents' minds. For him, it was immediately after he learned of Alice's difficult delivery that exploration of this possibility would have to be done.

Shortly after the Andersons had gone back to their home, Greg called to talk over this possibility. Robert was not sure they even had a lawyer at the time, but they certainly didn't have any idea how to go about finding one with whom to discuss a malpractice lawsuit.

Greg had never been one to keep hordes of acquaintances, but he always had several close friends, intensely loyal ones, always in touch with each other. His long-time best friend even up to the present is Robbie Ehrenberg. They had gone to nursery school together and grew up across the street from each other. Robbie's sister was a lawyer in Manhattan and she was the first person Robbie suggested that Greg contact. Robert wasn't sure how she knew who would be a good person to engage in Maneta or The City, but she had a lawyer in mind immediately. This attorney agreed that there were probably grounds for suing and he eventually guided them through the medical malpractice lawsuit process. The remarkable events surrounding the later parts of Alice's story eventually were handled by another legal group.

Greg and Carol had excellent advice throughout the ensuing lawsuit and their lawyers left no stone unturned in dealing with subsequent developments.

In the meantime, Greg and Carol continued to keep a record of events which later proved to be essential to the outcome of their legal struggle. Later on, knowing exactly what happened and when, made things easier for all concerned—Alice's parents as well as the lawyers on both sides.

Millie and Robert began to consider the possibility that they would be called to testify at trial.

Chapter 3

Medical Malpractice Pretrial Depositions

Deposition 1—Carol Anderson

On February 2, 1994, depositions of Greg and Carol began. Just the words, "Examination before trial . . . . " would be enough to frighten anyone. Carol went first to begin the legal proceedings with regard to the medical malpractice lawsuit being brought involving Alice's birth.

The depositions took place in the law offices of the Anderson's attorneys. Their lawyer was there, as was the lawyer for the defendant, Dr. Johnston. There were also several doctors present from Westside Hospital for Children, appearing for the defendant, as well as the malpractice company lawyer. This was the same medical malpractice company with which Dr. Anderson had his malpractice insurance.

Dr. Johnston's representative spoke first. Carol was informed that she would be able to have a question repeated or rephrased if necessary before she answered.

She was then asked about her date of birth, marriage, maiden name, how long she had lived at her current address as well as her previous addresses. Then about her education, which schools she had attended and their locations, her graduation dates and college career. She was admonished to answer questions only after the attorney had finished asking them for the convenience of the court reporter, because she tended to answer questions a bit too quickly. And the attorney conceded that he did tend to talk too fast, as well. (As if Carol were not nervous enough already—she should slow down, not the defendant's attorney!)

Carol then acknowledged that she had been an athletic trainer, but had no other medical or maternity training.

Next, she was asked to describe her work history—she was not then working—what her position was and what was her title. She indicated that, yes, she had handled medical malpractice claims and had undergone training to be able to do so. This was of great interest to the questioning lawyer. For the record, he "demanded" to have all written material connected in any way to the courses Carol took while she was a claims representative at the insurance company. Carol's lawyer wanted to know the reason for this and was informed that, since this was a malpractice case, such information might be relevant to her later testimony. Carol's lawyer said he would accept the "demand" if it was delivered in writing.

There followed an exhaustive description by Carol of her work, including reports, lawsuits, investigations, medical and damage reports and negotiated settlements with attorneys or claimants, in person as well as during progression to trial if one was needed.

Carol then had to explain what her job was early in her college career when she worked as a file clerk in the pediatric division of a large training hospital/medical school.

Then came Exhibits 1, 2 and 3. These were tax returns filed by Greg and Carol for several previous years. "And to your knowledge all the information in those tax returns is accurate?" asked the lawyer. It was.

Carol was then queried about her two children, Alice, and Gregory III, born after Alice's birth. There was interest in her son Gregory III's (G3's) age, health, possible congenital problems, birth defects. Once again Carol was admonished to slow down when giving her answers.

Alice and G3 had the same pediatricians.

Carol's family history was short since she had been adopted, had no knowledge of her natural parents or siblings. Carol's medical history became Exhibit 4. Even the color of the inks which had been used in filling out the forms was questioned! The black ink on the first page was Dr. Johnston's. Of course, the family medical history referred to Carol's adopted family.

Carol had never had any abnormal uterine bleeding. She had had her tonsils and adenoids removed as treatment for recurrent peritonsillar abscesses. She was to give the name of the surgeon. Even after this surgery, Carol continued to have abscesses in her oropharynx and was hospitalized at least once for this problem. She was required to name the hospital and the attending surgeon. Here a great deal of emphasis was put on the fact that the surgeon had been female; the reason was unclear. She was treated with antibiotics. She noted that she had had a D&C (dilatation and curettage) of her uterus under anesthesia for polyps, an abnormal Pap smear by Dr. Johnston long before Alice's birth and that she had undergone a caesarean section which had been planned from the start of her pregnancy with G3.

She noted springtime allergies including asthma and hay fever, most likely to tree pollen. These conditions had never been diagnosed officially or treated by a physician.

Almost every question Carol was asked was followed by the question, "Was that accurate at the time you checked it?" This referred to a list of medical questions that Carol had previously checked. This question was then followed by, "Is that still accurate through today?"

Naturally, there were questions about Carol's alcohol consumption. She was a "social" drinker, and quite adamantly denied ever having any alcohol during either of her pregnancies. She answered, "None whatsoever" to these queries.

She also had not had any caffeine during her pregnancy with Alice, and had never smoked at all. She also truthfully denied ever having marijuana or cocaine whether pregnant or not. She denied any allergies to medications.

During questioning, a problem arose over the name of a drug that Carol said she was taking presently. She had written something and then whited it out. It was difficult to read, but it appeared as if she had written "penicillin". She thought that she might have been on penicillin when she filled out the form either for her acne or for her tonsillitis, but obscured the entry because she couldn't remember accurately which antibiotic she was taking.

When told by the defendant's attorney that he would try to find out all the physicians that Carol had seen over the course of her life, her response was, "Oh, God!" (Given that one often cannot remember what one had for breakfast that day, this was an entirely appropriate response). The investigation of this question would include hospitals, clinics, such as her college medical facility, her dentists and her pediatricians. (An utterly impossible task and quite likely a useless one.)

Next Carol was asked about her contraceptive history. She had used only a diaphragm.

There followed a review of Carol's use of antibiotics, which seemingly were all penicillin relatives. She denied previous pneumonias, bronchitis, blood tests not related to hospitalization, and genetic testing. She said that she had never been told that there was any more risk than normal for birth defects in children that she might have.

Carol had chosen Dr. Johnston as her gynecologist when she came to Maneta and started going for her yearly exam about two years before her pregnancy with Alice. Dr. Johnston also did the previously mentioned D&C and removal of polyps. Carol then noted that what had been described as "excessive vaginal bleeding" was probably a heavy period which she was prone to have. She did not accept the word "excessive". She had never been treated for "heavy periods".

Here, it must be said that all of the questions Carol was asked about her pregnancy with Alice ought to have been asked. As will be seen, however, none of them had any bearing on the outcome of the pregnancy.

So then came questions about Carol's pregnancy with Alice. Yes, this was her first pregnancy. She noted that she had had one or two colds and a throat infection, which, interestingly, was treated by Dr. Johnston and not her regular medical doctor. She did not remember taking any other medication beyond the antibiotic Dr. Johnston prescribed and noted that she would not have taken any other medications, especially OTC ones without express permission from her obstetrician. She denied any other illnesses including stomach virus or "flu". She did take prenatal vitamins, but did not take any medications for her acne.

Carol then noted that she had had some vaginal bleeding very early in the pregnancy (the subject of the telephone call referred to previously in which she talked with Dr. Howell on Cape Cod.) She had performed a home pregnancy test which confirmed the pregnancy. The bleeding was "very, very light spotting". The bleeding produced brownish blood, not bright red blood, and occurred on one other day about two days later. It did not recur after that.

Carol also noted that she had a whitish vaginal discharge as the pregnancy proceeded. (This would be a normal development.) In addition to Dr. Howell, she also discussed the spotting with the obstetrician and the radiologist who performed the sonogram. This was explained as a possible twin pregnancy in which the second fetus had failed.

Carol also denied sexual intercourse during the last two weeks before Alice was born.

Carol was then asked to describe her visits with Dr. Johnston. During the pregnancy they varied little except that she initially saw him earlier than normal because of the spotting. She did remember one visit in detail just before she gave birth.

Normally, at a visit, Carol would be asked questions pertinent to the stage of the pregnancy, whether there were any problems or unexpected symptoms. An assistant would then take her vital statistics such as weight, blood pressure and a urine test. Other tests might also be done at that time. Then she would meet with Dr. Johnston. He did a vaginal exam at her first visit and at the final visit before Alice was born. Carol did not recall any other vaginal exams.

She was shown the sonograms, including the one which showed "the vanishing twin syndrome". This occurs when one of a set of twin fetuses apparently disappears from the uterus during pregnancy, usually resulting in a normal singleton pregnancy. The missing fetus spontaneously aborts so that it appears that the twin has vanished. It has been confirmed scientifically that the number of twin conceptions greatly out-numbers the total of actual twin births.

She described her last visit in detail. Greg had accompanied her. There was some discrepancy about the due date since Carol knew quite specifically when she had conceived. Greg had been out of town for several days on business at that time and been home for a specific number of days between two trips. Since Carol had had some early bleeding and since there was a question about her due date, an early ultrasound should perhaps have been done but was not. On the basis of history alone then, the doctor moved Carol's due date to a slightly earlier one, about a week earlier, June 7. Carol thought that this might be a reasonable date since her first due date was the middle to the end of June. She explained to Dr. Johnston that she thought this might be off by a week or two. She herself felt that early June would be the right time period.

At this last office visit, Carol's cervix was found to be two to three centimeters dilated and slightly effaced (the cervical edge was becoming flattened).

On the Sunday morning before Alice was born, very early, Carol awoke with uterine contractions. She and Greg timed the contractions—they were about five to seven minutes apart—and so Carol called the number the doctor had given her. She reached an answering service, explained the problem, and was told that Dr. Johnston was not on call that weekend and that one of his associates would get back to her.

When the covering doctor called, they discussed Carol's contractions and she was told to go to the hospital to have things checked out. She was at the hospital for about two hours. There had been no discharge of vaginal fluid.

Upon arrival at the Hospital for Children, Carol was placed in an examining room, blood pressure and a urine sample were taken and, Carol thought, a blood sample as well. Then she was hooked up to a fetal monitor for about 45 minutes, during which an internal exam was also done. A "doctor" and a "nurse" were present, but Carol was unacquainted with either. The attending obstetrician was called and suggested that Carol be up walking around to see if her contractions would speed up or become stronger. When nothing changed, she was again placed on the fetal monitor which also showed no change. At about 10 to 11 o'clock in the morning, Carol was sent home.

Up until then, nothing had happened that would be considered unusual in the care of a woman nearing delivery. Greg had been with Carol throughout.

Carol had previously had Dr. Johnston's permission to walk her regular walk after the first trimester and she went for a walk during the day after coming home from the hospital. She had a nap. In the evening after dinner, she and Greg went to their Lamaze class.

Carol's water broke at 2:00 am the next morning while she was sleeping. There was a gush of water which woke her instantly. She told her husband.

The fluid was colorless, and, when questioned more closely, Carol said that it was "maybe slightly pinkish, maybe." The defendant's attorney told her "not to guess." Carol responded that the fluid looked like what she had been told to expect it to look like. And she noted that she had not had any prior leaking of fluid. The mild contractions, off and on, did not change after her water broke. Then she spoke with the covering doctor again via the answering service. He may have teased her a bit, Carol said, about waking him up two nights in a row, but told her to go to the hospital once again. She arrived there before 6:00 am.

At this point, the hospital records indicated that Carol was having lower abdominal and back pain and that the contractions seemed to be coming from the back towards the front. Still, there was no severe pain. At no time had Carol experienced any vaginal bleeding.

Here there was a short exchange between lawyers. The Anderson's lawyer noted that Carol was testifying as to what she knew, not what the defendant's attorney was reading from the record.

Now, the hospital record showed that, upon admission, a list of symptoms showed that "spotting" had been crossed out and the word "bleeding" written in. Carol denied that she told anyone that she had been bleeding.

Then, Carol was asked about her and her husband's Lamaze classes. These were taken through the Lamaze Association in a private home. They had done this on the recommendation of a girlfriend of Carol's who felt she had benefitted from them. Carol could not just then recall the name of the instructor.

Quite abruptly and inexplicably, the next question to Carol was, "What physician delivered G3?" She did not remember his name, but knew that he was an associate of her current "OB-GYN". She had also seen another doctor associated with that office. At her first visit, immediately upon being introduced to one another, the doctor said, "Mrs. Anderson, you will be having a cesarean section." Clearly, her history was well known in the local obstetrical community. She also said that she had been seen in her college clinic by a gynecologist. What was the sudden interest in her gynecologists all about, Carol wondered, besides showing her to be confused about all the names from the past?

Then, it was back to the sore throats. Was she suffering from a sore throat when she went into labor with Alice? Did she feel sick in any way during the three days before she delivered Alice? Did she have stomach upset? Virus? Sore throat (again) or a cold? (These questions were probably meant to secure an explanation for Carol's high white blood cell count after delivery. It was an unsuccessful effort.)

The defendant's lawyer then began a review of Carol's testimony so far in the deposition. From then on reference was to Carol's second hospital admission. Once again repeat questions such as: Did Carol remember having blood drawn? What were the doctors' names? Carol remembered that, once again it was a female doctor, but not the same one she had seen the day before at her first visit.

Understandably, Carol did not remember specifics from her conversations at this time, but she did remember being told that she was going to be kept in the hospital this time. She reaffirmed that her labor was still "desultory" after her water broke. After she had had an internal exam in one room she was taken to a "birthing room". In the birthing room, Greg and Carol tried to make themselves as comfortable as possible. There was one nurse who was present from time to time, and then at least two other nurses were assigned to watch over things. Carol asked if she could be monitored by the external fetal monitor for about fifteen minutes and then be able to walk around.

About 10:00 am Dr. Johnston appeared in the birthing room. Carol noted that her contractions were still relatively mild and the doctor said that he might have to augment labor. He also indicated that Carol should walk around, place hot packs on her breasts and have a hot shower. This was Carol's first encounter with Dr. Johnston that day. He did not examine Carol in any way.

Much later in the day, a female hospital resident appeared. Carol did not remember whether she had seen this person before. Carol recalled that an internal exam "might possibly" have been done then. She was only about four centimeters dilated at that time. Eventually the contractions began to be stronger and Carol was unable to continue walking around. According to the monitor which had been placed again, the baby's heart rate was strong and things seemed to be going well. While Carol had been walking around, presumably in the hallway, the fetal monitor was being used about 15 minutes out of every hour. Eventually, the monitor was turned on continuously.

Greg was with Carol the entire day. They went through the Lamaze breathing exercises.

Eventually, probably in the early afternoon, an epidural was performed. This was apparently done by an OB-GYN resident. Nowadays, it would be very unusual for a resident to be doing epidural anesthesia. However, by this time Carol was six centimeters dilated. All the internal exams were done by a physician. The latest exam was done by a female doctor, but Carol was not sure if she was the same one who had attended to her earlier. The epidural was done because Carol was having a great deal of back pain unrelieved by breathing exercises, position changes, etc.

The next person to appear was an anesthesiologist. Carol remembered little of this doctor when asked, such as whether he had a beard or not! Carol explained that she was worried that she would move during a contraction while the epidural anesthesia was being administered. All in attendance reassured her. Carol said that she "probably" gave consent for the epidural, but she did not recall having the risks or alternatives to the procedure being explained to her. The epidural eventually provided Carol with some alleviation of her back pain.

She continued to experience vaginal pressure. She thought the epidural was given about 4:00 pm. This, of course, ought to have been clear in the hospital record.

Then Carol was asked about anyone else she remembered coming in to see her. She recalled speaking with the nurse who came in to help with the breathing technique that Greg and Carol had learned. This nurse recommended an anesthetic medicine for pain relief and this was given to Carol about 2:00 pm. (The drug was Nubain, an analgesic narcotic commonly used for simple surgeries and during labor, but rarely administered after a successful epidural. While not relieving pain, it does lessen pain perception making the pain more tolerable.) Carol was unsure by whose authority the Nubain was administered, but it did help temporarily.

When asked with whom else she talked, Carol mentioned that, during her walks earlier, there were comments from the staff about how busy it was getting at that time in the obstetric section of the hospital.

Carol started "pushing" at about 6:00 pm. Up until then there had been other house staff physicians in her room from time to time, but not Dr. Johnston.

In the time following the epidural, Carol remembered discussing Alice's heart rate which was being observed on the fetal monitor. Then the heart rate recording suddenly stopped. Greg and Carol both noticed this and Greg went to get a nurse or a doctor. No one came back to the room with Greg, and it was a significantly long time before someone from the hospital came into the room. Carol did not know who came into the room, looked at the monitor and said that it was not picking up a heart rate. An attempt was made to reposition the monitoring strips placed on Carol's abdomen. Eventually, the fetus' heart rate was picked up again, only to disappear shortly thereafter. Greg went to report this.

Carol was repeatedly questioned about which medical personnel were in and out of her room. She was supposed remember all these people by name!

Even Greg tried to reposition the monitoring strips. Then someone went to call Dr. Johnston. This was about 5:00 pm. He showed up at about 6:00 pm, the second time Carol had seen him during the day. Also about 6:00 pm an internal monitor was put on the baby.

(Internal fetal monitoring is used for high risk births or for normal births when the birth team is having trouble keeping the baby on the external monitor or the baby's reaction does not look good. The mother's bag of waters must be broken, which Carol's was, by now about 14 hours previously. In this procedure, a fetal scalp electrode is placed by screwing a tiny wire into the top layers of the baby's scalp. This method does not use ultra sound and thus is more accurate than the external monitor.)

And now, the attendants were unable to get this mechanism to operate correctly. The electrodes were disconnected and someone went to get new ones. Eventually, Dr. Johnston was able to place a functioning internal monitor on the baby.

Between 4:00 and 6:00 pm, Carol also spoke with someone about the increasing vaginal pressure she was experiencing with the contractions. An anesthesiologist was to come to check on Carol, presumably about the epidural, but no one ever came. (An anesthesiologist did come back into the birthing room after Alice was born to check the epidural. At that time, he apologized for not checking on Carol prior to Alice's birth. He indicated that he had done several C-sections that evening. Eventually, a day later, another anesthesiologist came by the room to check on any side effects from the epidural.) Carol's labor then progressed steadily, gradually. Her cervix was becoming satisfactorily dilated and Dr. Johnston said that it was time for Carol to "push". Carol did not know if she was fully dilated. When Carol was asked if Dr. Johnston remained with her from the time she started pushing through the birth of the baby, she said, "No." Carol's husband and the nurse were with Carol now, while she was pushing.

Eventually, Dr. Johnston did return to the birthing room and instructed Carol on the technique she should use to push. She was to do Valsalva maneuvers when pushing. (Valsalva breathing methods consist of trying to exhale forcibly through a closed windpipe so that no air exits through the mouth or nose.)

Alice was delivered at 8:05 pm. There followed intense questioning about the time period between 6:00 and 8:00 pm. Carol did not recall another conversation with Dr. Johnston or other doctors. She remained in the birthing room during this entire time and Alice was delivered there. Carol did not remember specific conversations she had during this period. She said that she badly wanted a Coca Cola. Greg was giving her ice chips. She did not recall hearing anything about a forceps delivery or anything being said about an anesthesiologist during this period of time. Just before Alice was born, Dr. Johnston was in the room trying to help the baby to be born while Carol was pushing. She did not recall any other conversations with personnel at that time.

Carol realized that the baby's head was not crowning. (Crowning refers to the time when the widest part of the baby's head, or its crown, is emerging from the vagina. Normally part of the forehead to the eyebrows and the back of the baby's head can be clearly seen.)

Carol did not recall what was said at the time. Soon, Alice's head was finally crowning. Carol did realize that an episiotomy was going to be performed. (An episiotomy is a surgical incision made in the area between the vagina and the anus, the perineum, to expand the opening of the vagina to prevent tearing there during the delivery of the baby.) A local anesthetic was administered by needle, which Carol noted "freaked me out" even though an effective epidural should obviate the need for an episiotomy. Then Alice was born, with great relief for Carol. She remembers touching the baby and being told that she had had a girl. Right then Carol did not recall hearing anything said about the condition of the baby.

Then the defendant's lawyer asked if there was a point in time when Carol learned that the baby had some problems. She answered that there was.

Baby Alice had been handed into the care of the intensive pediatric care nursing team while Dr. Johnston continued completing the delivery of the placenta and suturing the episiotomy. Carol remembered hearing a communication over the PA system that said something about the umbilical cord pH, a measure of the acidity or alkalinity of the blood. At this point, Dr. Johnston became very upset and said, "What? Repeat that!" loudly into the speaker system. The pH number was 6.8. Carol knew that that was not normal.

(Infants with an umbilical cord pH of less than 7.00 are at risk of manifesting hypoxic ischemic encephalopathy and subsequent neurological dysfunction. This, in essence, means that the baby's brain has suffered a lack of oxygen and lack of blood supply causing brain damage which often results in cerebral palsy.)

Carol was able to observe the nurses working on Alice. With the presence of the intensive pediatric care group, she knew something thing was wrong. Carol described Alice as unresponsive, lying on the table in the bright lights and "she was just a rag doll, floppy". Then the baby was whisked off to the pediatric intensive care unit.

Carol had no further conversation with the obstetrician at that time. Carol remembered his talking about a vacuum extractor, but she did not know the importance of this. The doctor commented that he had used the correct extractor. (Vacuum extractors have essentially replaced forceps in vaginal deliveries because they cause fewer neonatal scalp injuries. However, since extractors can cause neonatal injury as well, they must be used only when indicated such as with a non-reassuring fetal heart tracing or failing satisfactory progress in advanced labor.)

During the remainder of her stay in the hospital, Carol had several conversations with Dr. Johnston about Alice's birth and her condition.

The morning after Alice's birth, Dr. Johnston came into Carol's room. By that time Carol was being given antibiotics. He told her that she was having the medication because her white blood cell count was elevated (it was 22,000, a sign of infection—normal would be about 5-10,000).

The doctor told the new mother and father that Alice was having seizures. Coming after they had been told that the baby was doing well, this comment was frightening.

He also said that he had thought about doing a caesarian section, but, obviously, had decided against it. He did not tell Carol why he had decided against the C-section.

(Of course, it is impossible to say for sure, but Alice may have been born a perfectly normal baby had he done a C-section. While the number of C-sections is increasing dramatically at present, now around 30% and climbing, there was reluctance during the time period when Alice was born for obstetricians to have high rates of C-section on their record, a level of 5% being acceptable. Hospital medical boards did not approve of high C-section percentage rates.)

Then, the obstetrician examined Carol's episiotomy and checked her chart.

The next day, Dr. Johnston appeared again. Carol's white blood count was coming down. He did not mention Alice's condition. The following day Carol and he discussed post-partum instructions: what Carol's care should be at home where she was to continue the antibiotics and that he would see her in six weeks for her post-partum visit. Once again there was no discussion of Alice or how she was doing.

(Normally, one would think that there would be a good bit of discussion/banter about the new baby. Was the doctor worried now about what would transpire legally in the near future? For instance, there is no mention of a neonatologist being present.)

During her first month at home, Carol developed breast discomfort. She was not breast feeding, but was breast pumping in order to take her milk to Alice in the hospital. She was also running a temperature. At that time, while Carol was in the intensive care nursery, her mother, Helga, called Dr. Johnston. He said that if she would go to the delivery suite in the hospital one of the doctors there would see her. Helga and the doctor did not discuss Alice at all. A little after this, Carol developed a total body rash and discussed that with Dr. Johnston. He referred her to a dermatologist who decided that the rash was due to "hormones" and "stress", but did not name a specific cause for the rash nor specifically treat it.

Then, six weeks after the delivery, Carol saw Dr. Johnston for the last time at her post-partum visit. He examined her and pronounced her nicely recovered. He asked her how Alice was doing, finally.

By that time, Alice was home from the hospital and Carol thought that Alice was doing everything a six-week old baby should be doing at that point. Carol was alone at this visit and there was no further conversation about Alice.

The defendant's attorney then wanted to know if, other than her attorney, anyone had ever said anything that was critical of Dr. Johnston's care, mentioning things that the obstetrician may have done wrong. Carol's attorney asked for clarification of this question for Carol who did not understand what was meant by it.

Carol, somewhat enlightened now, said that yes, she had had numerous discussions with her family members about what had happened. Had any physician ever said anything along those lines? Carol's reply was, "I would have to say yes". She identified her father-in-law, agreeing with the questioner that he was a physician. That would be Dr. Anderson, of course, who is an allergist/immunologist. A conversation with one of

Alice's intensive care nurses regarding taking legal action about what had happened at Alice's birth did take place, as, for example, "pursuing a law suit". The nurse did not elaborate or directly criticize the hospital or the doctor, but she did imply that the matter should be looked into. There were no comments from other physicians, nurses or medical professionals.

The questioning abruptly turned to whether Alice had been seen at Westside Hospital for Children. She had been seen there as well as at the Rehabilitation Center. Then Carol needed to recite a long list of the clinics and doctors whom Alice had seen up to then. These included a pediatric clinic and The Feeding Clinic, as well as the Colonial Education Program. Alice had also seen a private pediatrician and a dentist.

At two months of age, Alice appeared to choke on formula. Since, at the time, they were staying with Henry and Helga, Carol's parents, a trip to a local clinic seemed necessary. There, Alice was declared to be "fine".

Carol was then asked about Alice's seizures. They had stopped about four days after her birth and had not recurred, to Carol's knowledge.

Carol was then asked what she understood to be Alice's health problems at the present time. She replied, "Moderate to severe cerebral palsy and microcephaly". She went on to say that the cerebral palsy would cause her physical handicaps and that microcephaly was a "small head". She noted, also, that Alice was severely developmentally delayed. When asked to elaborate, Carol noted that Alice did not roll over, did not sit up, was still bottle fed, and did not talk. Her care was what a three month old would require. Alice was now two years and eight months old.

Questions followed again about Carol's employment. She was not then employed, having last worked up to mid-January, 1992. Carol had gone back to work five months after Alice was born and continued to work until January of the following year.

Her son, Gregory III, was born in April of 1993.

When asked why she had quit working in January, 1992, Carol replied, "It got to be too much taking care of Alice, trying to get her to her various clinics and doctors' appointments and I just couldn't continue working and managing to do all that and, you know, doing my best at work." Carol then named the baby sitter she had employed for Alice.

The defendant's attorney asked Carol about the Bill of Particulars which Greg and Carol had signed. This bill refers to a number of injuries and health problems that Alice suffered from.

What did "severe perinatal asphyxia" mean to Carol? That meant Alice had insufficient oxygen around the time of or during her birth. Next was "fetal distress". Carol responded that while "in utero" or while being delivered, Alice had distress due to lack of oxygen. Breathing trouble after being delivered also was contributory. Then, "severe metabolic acidosis". (By now Carol might have been a third year medical student!) That meant, to Carol, that at birth, Alice's metabolism was abnormal and was associated with the abnormal pH levels. Carol did not know what "sepsis" meant. That would be a generalized, blood-borne infection. By "impaired mental development" Carol responded that, as a result of Alice's brain damage at birth, her cognitive development was severely retarded. Alice's pediatricians and neurologists had explained that to Carol. Carol was asked about "stunted growth". Carol understood that Alice would be shorter than she would have been normally largely because she does not bear weight as by standing up. Carol then noted that Alice's gross and fine motor skills were totally impaired.

Alice also had a "lazy eye" which had been corrected about four months prior to this questioning. Her sight in that eye at that time appeared to be impaired. Hearing impairment was not definitely present largely because of the difficulty in testing the child for that. She also had profoundly impaired speech development—Alice made sounds but did not converse or talk. Also, Alice could not chew and could not swallow normally. She was unable to drink from a Sippy-cup.

Then there was "muscular rigidity and excessive muscle tone". Carol replied that Alice was "spastic". Carol then described the Anderson's efforts to alleviate the stiffness. They included her passive muscle stretching exercises daily so that Alice's bones, such as her hip bones, would remain in alignment. How about "impaired renal function"? Carol knew that after the baby had been born there was some damage to the kidneys, but that did improve. And then, "hypoxic ischemic encephalopathy". At this point, the Anderson's lawyer indicated to Carol, in a rebuke to the opposing attorney, that she was not being asked to testify as a medical expert.

Finally, this part of the questioning was over and the discussion moved on to which doctors, working where, did what. The list was a long one.

Carol was asked if a nurse was with her in the birthing room from 4:00 pm until Alice was born, and if the nurse did leave the room from time to time. She was, in fact, out of the room more than she was in it with Carol. Sometimes, Carol thought, the nurse reviewed the monitoring strip.

Dr. Johnston came to Carol's room between 6:00 pm and the time the baby was born. When he returned nearer to the time of the delivery, Carol was already pushing. Carol did not know how close that was to the delivery. Eventually, Dr. Johnston came into the room and stayed there continuously until the baby was born. Carol did not remember just when this was nor, of course, how many times she had pushed. Carol noted that she was not paying much attention to how much time had elapsed, how many times she pushed or just when the doctor was present. She was, after all, in labor. Carol was unwilling to guess at these questions and Carol's lawyer had urged her not to guess.

Carol discussed the baby's birth with nurses after Alice's delivery. It seemed that every nurse who came to care for Carol would ask if she had been down to the intensive care nursery and how the baby was doing. Carol was getting her information from the intensive care unit. Carol had seen the baby for a quick glance just as Alice was being transferred to the nursery.

Then, when Carol was being wheeled to her room after the delivery, a man who, Carol thought, might be a doctor, stopped the transfer to tell Carol what was going on. He noted that Alice was as stable as they could get her and that she was in serious condition. Shortly thereafter, Carol did go into the intensive care nursery to see Alice as the nurses were working on her. They had little new information and mainly tried to cheer Carol up a bit.

The following morning, the Andersons called down to the nursery and talked with Alice's primary care nurse. By that time, Alice's condition was stable and she had been able to suck. This news cheered Carol and Greg immensely. Alice was going to be all right.

But then, Dr. Johnston appeared and told Carol and Greg that Alice was having seizures. In Neonatal Intensive Care, the nurses tried to explain what was being done for Alice, what her condition was and to describe what all the "things" that were attached to her were for. Carol was witness to the seizures. Alice had had an EEG (electroencephalograph) and a spinal tap. She was being given the same antibiotics that Carol was receiving. And, a developmental pediatrician had been called in. Alice's prognosis at this point was for mild to moderate disability due to lack of oxygen to her brain, but that the baby would live.

A theme throughout all this questioning was whether or not Carol had spoken to any staff and what those people had said. She was asked repeatedly about this.

Information was coming to the Andersons from the physicians, the resident staff in the nursery and the nurses. After Carol left the hospital she did not discuss her care during labor and delivery with anyone. No one ever criticized the care she received during her labor and delivery. The only criticism she heard came from Dr. Anderson, her father-in-law. Dr. Anderson said that "it shouldn't have happened" with regard to Alice's abnormal birth. Dr. Anderson visited early and talked to one of the doctors. Carol could not remember his criticizing anything specific about Carol's care. Carol did recall that Dr. Anderson had suggested that a C-section should have been done. He was able to put circumstances and activities into layman's terms for his children, explaining what the physician he had talked with had said. There had been a definite problem that hadn't been addressed, but nothing more specific. At no time did Dr. Anderson speak with Dr. Johnston.

Next, Carol was asked what things Alice could do, having explained what she could not do.

She could not grab onto things. She did make "D", "B" and "G" sounds occasionally. She seemed quite well. She had a good range of motion of her head and could hold her head up. Some ideas could be gotten across to her, not the other way around. For example: whether she wants juice, or to eat. She seemed to recognize some people's voices. She was uncomfortable and somewhat fearful around strangers, but she appeared comfortable with several women who come to care for her from respite services. This is not paid service. Occasionally hired babysitters cared for Alice, as well.

Alice could be spoon-fed. All of her food had to be pureed in a food processor—including soups. This continued throughout her life. But her diet was largely the same as the rest of the family. Alice did not require supplemental nutrition.

She had trouble even taking fluids from a bottle because the thinner liquids caused her to choke. Milk was better because it was thicker.

Alice's next medical appointments were to be with an orthopedic surgeon, ophthalmologist for follow-up on surgery to correct Alice's "lazy eye", and neurologist. Alice had no other scheduled surgeries. At that time, no one anticipated improvement in Alice's other skills.

The orthopedic surgeon saw Alice every six months and the neurologist every year. Alice saw her pediatricians on a yearly basis, as well and, in the meantime, a nurse-practitioner because of Alice's chronic constipation.

There was no prognosis from the orthopedist. The neurologist noted that, because the growth of Alice's head was slowing down, her prognosis for neurologic improvement wasn't good. The pediatricians simply followed Alice without commenting on prognoses.

The developmental pediatrician had told the Andersons that Alice had moderate to severe cerebral palsy that she was mentally retarded and was severely developmentally delayed. The Andersons did plan to continue to keep Alice at home with them.

Then it was back to Dr. Anderson. Had he ever spoken with Dr. Johnston? He had not. On the other hand, Mrs. Anderson, Millie, spoke with him, as mentioned, in the hallway. Millie had also overheard Dr. Johnston telling the Andersons that he had considered doing a C-section. (Since Alice's birth, the rate of cesarean births has been increasing. Associated with an increased rate of primary cesarean birth, indications may be subjective such as non-reassuring fetal heart tracing status or arrest of dilation, arrest of descent and malpresentation. Also included is maternal request. By these accounts, cesarean delivery may have been indicated in Alice's case. Efforts to reduce the increasing cesarean rate included increased provider accountability for the decision to perform cesarean delivery at the practice, departmental, hospital or state level. Journal reference: Obstet Gynecol, 2011; 1:29-38)

A notebook (Exhibit 5) was asked about. This was a diary that Carol and Greg had kept following Alice's birth. There followed an utterly nonsensical discussion among the lawyers as to how many pages were in the diary; who wrote what on which side of each page and how the counting was done.

Finally, it was agreed that there were 22 handwritten pages in the journal. The handwriting was Greg's. Information included out-of-pocket expenses. At the very end there was a handwritten note stapled to the page, written by Millie. Then, an agreement was reached that the Andersons could be recalled to testify about findings in the diary.

There were some final questions for Carol. Had she planned to return to work after Alice's birth? Yes, full-time. Had a special chair been purchased for Alice? Yes, a chair to give Alice additional support while she was eating. A traditional high chair was not an option since Alice was unable to sit up on her own. For some inexplicable reason, Carol was asked to compare G3's development with Alice's. The contrast was profound, Gregory III being an entirely normal baby.

Deposition 2—Greg Anderson

The questioning of Greg began with the defendant's attorney. The same rules applied as had with Carol

Vital statistics came first, such as date of birth, number of marriages, number of children besides Alice and G3. Greg answered more questions about when and where he had graduated from college, where he went to high school and when he had graduated. He was asked about post-graduate training, and where he had obtained his Master of Arts degree, in which discipline and when. Greg noted that he was currently employed with an environmental consulting firm and that he dealt mainly with groundwater issues. Which other firms had he worked for were discussed and the fact that Greg ran the campus pizza shop where he had gone to college. And, prior to that, he had been employed as a house painter. The lawyer was looking for something in Greg's background, such as a chemical exposure, which might have affected Alice's condition.

Greg was asked if he had had any medical or paramedical training. He had had standard CPR and first aid training, only.

Then Greg's family history became the topic, since Carol, having been adopted, was not able to supply answers to family history questions. Greg had two brothers, one older, Robert, Jr. and one younger, Andrew. He also had an older sister, Joyce. Did anyone in his family ever suffer from any genetic or birth disorders? Greg knew that there were two second cousins on his father's side who had had Batten's Disease. Greg was unaware of what this disease was except that it was a genetic disorder, and could give no more information about it. (Batten's disease is a fatal, progressive, inherited disorder of the nervous system that begins in childhood, usually between the ages of five and ten.) Then the lawyer asked how Greg knew that they had had some sort of disorder. "They're deceased," he replied. He was asked to supply the parents' name, which he did.

Greg did not know of any other examples of cerebral palsy in his family, or of breathing disorders, learning disabilities or mental retardation. Greg himself had never been hospitalized and had not had any extraordinary health problems. He denied genetic or blood testing.

Greg then was asked how often he accompanied Carol on her visits to Dr. Johnston prior to Alice's birth. These were in the last month of Carol's pregnancy. Greg had no communication with Dr. Johnston except for the doctor's demonstration of his examination of Carol and the instruments he used as well as the degree of dilatation and effacement there was at the last office visit.

Greg was also with Carol during her hospital visits prior to Alice's birth. At the first visit everything Greg noted was essentially in agreement with Carol's testimony. Greg denied hearing any conversations at the first hospital visit that Carol had not already mentioned. At home after that visit, there were no conversations with doctors

Greg was asked about what time Carol told him that her waters broke. "About 1:00 or 2:00 o'clock in the morning," he said. They then called the doctor, but someone other than Dr. Johnston called back. The lawyer then wanted to know if Greg knew whether or not Carol was having any vaginal bleeding on the morning she was admitted to the hospital. He denied knowing that. He said that when he changed the bed sheets after Carol's water broke there was no blood or meconium on the sheets. (Meconium is a tar-like substance lining a fetus's intestines during pregnancy. The substance is not obvious until the baby's bowel movement after birth. If meconium is present during labor and birth it may be a sign of fetal distress and the baby would be monitored more closely than usual)

Greg noted that he spoke with Dr. Johnston in mid-morning after Carol was admitted. The doctor inquired what had taken place the day before. He was basically checking up on how Carol was doing and what point had been reached in Carol's labor.

Greg saw Dr. Johnston again in the evening. Before that, during the day, he spoke with a nurse examining Carol who recommended Nubain and then, since the pain was not alleviated, Dr. Johnston discussed an epidural with Carol and Greg.

The anesthesiologist came, looked at Carol's chart, and discussed the procedure with the Andersons. Greg did not remember the doctor telling them about the risks of an epidural. Since Greg was not allowed to be present during the administration of the epidural, he had little information to offer the attorney. (An epidural is not likely to increase the need for a C-section. However, significant low blood pressure, hypotension, can occur and fetal heart rate deceleration and fetal distress have been noted following epidurals. Maternal convulsions and loss of consciousness can occur. There can be bleeding into the spinal cord and headache. Infection at the injection site can occur as well as back pain. Uterine contractions can become less frequent and weaker. Epidurals sometimes result in an increased use of forceps or vacuum extractions as compared with non-medicated women. Since local anesthetics rapidly cross the placenta, they can result in various degrees of maternal, fetal and neonatal toxicity.)

Then Greg described his listening to the anesthesiologist saying that the pump to the mechanical syringe was empty when it should have been full. Greg did not know if anyone ever refilled the pump. When asked repeatedly, Greg finally estimated at about what time he spoke to the anesthesiologist.

Greg denied hearing any mention by Dr. Johnston about the looming delivery upon the doctor's arrival in the birthing room. He did ask Greg to do certain things to help Carol out during her labor such as giving her ice chips but not too many of them. After that, Dr. Johnston peered frequently at the fetal monitor screen. Dr. Johnston apparently knew at this point that he would "have to move the baby's head around to assist in the delivery".

Greg noted that Dr. Johnston was absent from the birthing room several times up until the delivery, but Greg did not recall for how long at a time. No one at this time said anything about Carol's being ready to deliver the baby.

Then, Greg gave a long description of the delivery. Carol had been pushing for two hours. It seemed as though the baby could not or did not fit into the birth canal. Dr. Johnston spent quite some time trying to turn the baby's head in the birth canal. When asked if he could see whether Dr. Johnston had an instrument in his hand, Greg explained where everyone was placed around Carol and then he said, "I saw what he was doing. What I could see, I could see, what I couldn't see, I couldn't see. I knew that the doctor was trying to maneuver the baby's head so as to assist in the birth." Here it seems that Greg was becoming a bit impatient with the questioning, perhaps because he knew he was going to have to relive Alice's birth.

Greg saw the baby's head crown, so he knew from the classes he and Carol had taken that Alice was ready to be delivered. Nurses from the neonatal intensive care unit were there with the warmed bed. Greg was told to hurry up and cut the cord. He knew by now that Alice was a girl. She was blue, very discolored. Greg thought they were respirating her by then, with a respirator bag on her face. His recollection of the talk related to the pH was the same as Carol's.

Greg noted that Dr. Johnston came into the birthing room after residents had done an internal exam on Carol and they had called him.

The morning following the birth, Carol, Greg and Dr. Johnston spoke. That was when they learned that Alice was having seizures, but that she was "fine" and Carol was doing well so soon after the delivery. Neither of these remarks proved to be true.

Other communications with Dr. Johnston were noted to be the same as Carol had reported. Greg said that he encountered Dr. Johnston once in the hospital parking lot, but that no conversation between them took place. Greg repeated that no one beside his father, Dr. Anderson, had spoken about the obstetrician. No other hospital personnel of any sort had spoken to Greg about Dr. Johnston.

Greg then noted that he had read only his notes (Exhibit 5) in preparation for the current questioning. He said that he had kept the diary and he verified the testimony with regard to the diary that Carol had given.

The next questioner was, again, the attorney representing the medical malpractice carrier for the doctors and the hospital.

Greg testified that he had not had any conversations with the hospital's staff that pertained specifically to the hospital or to Alice's care. When asked if his father, Dr. Anderson, in any way criticized Alice's care, he responded that the care was not what his father saw as proper, but did not say what proper care was, in his father's opinion. Greg noted that he never had an in-depth conversation with Dr. Anderson regarding the care of Alice after her birth at the hospital.

Greg was then pressed to reveal any conversations he might have had or overheard which differed from Carol's recalling of them. When Carol asked Greg to go find someone to check the fetal monitor, he asked if someone could please come to check it out. This was after the epidural was placed. Greg seemed to know more about the monitor than the questioner.

When asked if Greg recalled whether there was a digital indication of the fetal heart rate at that time, Greg asked if they were now talking about the LED screen or the graphical display. The questioner wondered if they were both on the monitor and Greg replied that they were. Greg noted that he could see the paper tracings of the heart, as well a numerical display. Greg noted that there was no reading on one or the other or both of the displays. He also noted that here was an audible display which was also in the mixture.

Apparently, no one showed up immediately after Greg's request for help, but did come within half an hour. The time now was just after Carol returned from receiving the epidural. Greg was unsure if this was the first time he had not heard the audible record. When Greg explained that he did not know how a fetal monitor actually works, not being trained in that, the questioner interrupted saying that she was not asking him about the workings of the monitor.

There followed unrelenting questioning about when Greg went to the nurses' station, who was there, what sex they were, what their names were, even what they looked like and, of all things, what their race was. When Greg returned to Carol, there was still no signal on the monitor that told Greg that there was a heartbeat. There did seem to be some intermittent audible beats from the machine. Greg noted that there were two external sensors wrapped around Carol's waist this time.

Eventually, a female doctor showed up at Carol's bedside. She and a nurse were able to begin to get a record from the monitor again and announced that they were going to call Dr. Johnston to let him know what the monitor was telling them. Who said that Dr. Johnston was being called? Greg's reply was that he was paying attention to his wife and not to who was talking in the room. He did remember someone saying that Dr. Johnston would be told about the rapid decelerations in the fetal heart beat.

Greg then explained that two residents, both female, one black, one white, and a nurse were discussing the tracings on the fetal monitor in the doorway to the room. During the discussion, "rapid deceleration" was mentioned and, overall, the conversation took on an "air of urgency". They came back into the room and told the Andersons that Dr. Johnston was being called. At the time, no one explained what the term "rapid decelerations" meant to Greg or Carol. At an earlier time, however, a nurse had explained what the fetal monitoring tracings meant, and the Andersons had had some understanding of this from the birthing classes they had attended. This is rather complicated obstetrical stuff and Greg and Carol really had very little understanding of it especially with regard to "decelerations".

When Dr. Johnston was called, all medical personnel left the birthing room. When a doctor or nurse returned, the Andersons were told that Dr. Johnston would be there shortly and delivery would proceed from there.

In all, Greg had gone to the nurses' station two or three times to let them know that the monitor was not working the way it ought to be or at least, to explain that there were no readings being shown. Each time staff members came in and adjusted sensors strapped to Carol's abdomen. Greg then made at least two more trips to the nurses' station whereupon the staff responded more urgently, giving Carol oxygen and changing her position and attempting to re-place the monitor electrodes. Finally, as noted above, a resident doctor attempted to attach an internal monitor. The resident doctor was a female, Greg remembered, but, when Dr. Johnston arrived, the monitor once again was not functioning.

Now, Greg was asked to reiterate his lack of understanding of the operation and/or function of the fetal monitor.

The hospital's insurance attorney then insisted on knowing who was in Carol's room from 6:00 pm until 8:05 pm Greg remembered that no one was there with them the whole time, but that Dr. Johnston was occasionally there-"(with) all his comings and goings".

Then followed a long review of whether and to whom Greg had spoken following Alice's delivery. His testimony reflected Carol's testimony exactly. The stress here was upon what anyone might have said about the delivery. The attorney made a point of noting that the Andersons had taken Alice back to be seen at a different clinic, but at the same hospital where Alice's delivery had taken place.

The defendant's attorney then began re-examination of Greg. Greg was asked how long it took for Dr. Johnston to arrive in the birthing room after he had been called. The estimate was one hour. Then Greg was shown his tax returns just as Carol had been shown the returns. Greg confirmed that these were his returns and that the information on each of them was accurate. Greg was asked if he had anything to add to Carol's testimony about Alice's hospital, clinic and doctor visits. Greg verified that no conversations had taken place with staff members or physicians about Alice's current condition and prognosis other than already described by Carol.

The Anderson's attorney then verified Greg's testimony that, prior to Alice's birth, no one indicated to her parents that there were any potential problems or any concerns about her birth. Nor was there any explanation as to why the intensive care nursery staff was present in the room prior to Alice's birth.

Financial concerns were now addressed. "How have you been affected financially?" Greg was asked. He responded that losing Carol's entire income resulted in a 45% decrease in their income. They had had to refinance their home and did not roll over Greg's 401K account. They put off buying a second vehicle, having Carol use public transportation during the short time she went back to work after Alice was born.

After all of this preparatory work, the Anderson's and their lawyers decided to include the hospital in the lawsuit. Somewhere along the line, Alice's fetal monitoring record had disappeared from her chart. After the hospital became involved with the lawsuit, her monitoring record mysteriously reappeared in her chart. (Not only is it impermissible to make changes in a chart without careful documentation, reappearance of missing information can be fatal to a defendant's lawsuit. In addition, while the elder Andersons were prepared to have to testify in court, most if not all of the medical house staff who had attended to Alice had dispersed all over the country, more often than not very far away. Getting them together to testify would be a huge problem.)

In any case, these two factors caused the doctor and the hospital to capitulate immediately. Thus, finally, all that needed to be determined was the amount of compensation Alice would receive and how it would be distributed. The Andersons would not consider settling immediately, while their attorneys were picking a jury. They were given several offers in the few weeks prior to trial, but the Andersons felt they weren't enough for Alice's care. Even the judge involved was encouraging settlement, but they held out for a specific number which came from some of the experts their attorney had hired who estimated the cost of her care. Because they would have to be in court during a trial they had asked several family members to come and help them with Alice. But then the law suit was settled just before the actual trial started. The State had recently passed laws prohibiting acquisition of lump sum payments in cases like Alice's. Her award included monthly payments of several thousand dollars until she reached 21 years of age and then increased dramatically per month thereafter until her death. This presumed that Alice would need constant care either at home or if she was eventually institutionalized. Cost of living increases would be added. Payment would continue for life. Since Alice was basically healthy except for her CP, her life span could be normal or even longer.

Greg and Carol were granted control of Alice's estate and distributions from it. They were required to account for all of Alice's expenses on a monthly basis. All of her needs would be covered; these included payment to Carol for the extra time Alice's disabilities required her to provide care above and beyond that which would be necessary for a normal child.

An offshoot of the award was that Alice would not be able to inherit. Her grandparents sadly rearranged their wills to reflect this. Millie felt badly since she did have some jewelry of her own and from her family which she wanted eventually to give to the grandchildren. She finally decided to gift Alice a gold pin with sapphires and diamonds. She felt that Alice could wear this whenever she got "dolled up" and that it would be unlikely to disappear in the way that a ring or necklace might.

Chapter 4

Life with Alice

Alice had severe cerebral palsy (CP). CP may be classified as a wide range of disabilities from mild to profoundly severe. The disability is unique to each individual, i.e. CP affects the muscle control of each individual differently. In Alice's case, her muscle function was controlled by primitive reflexes as well as being affected by high tone or spasticity. The tone impacted her upper body more than her legs. Her tone could change from day to day, from morning to night or even from moment to moment. If she was tired, ill, upset or even extremely happy there might be an effect on what she could do at any given moment.

The Baclofen Pump

With this in mind, the Andersons and their doctors decided to try an Intrathecal Baclofen Pump (ITP). All had been following the research and success of the therapy on the internet for several years. ITP therapy involves a small hockey puck-shaped pump placed under Alice's skin near her hip. A tube from the pump to her spine delivered Baclofen directly into the intrathecal or intraspinal cavity of her spine. Where anatomically the dose is delivered depends on what issues one is trying to resolve. Because Alice's spasticity affected her upper body and arms so greatly, the tubing was placed as high as Alice's neurosurgeon could get it so her upper body would experience some relief.

While Alice was still in school, with Mary Tanner as her teacher, she received her Baclofen Pump. The Andersons had been following research for several years about various treatments to help kids with cerebral palsy such as Botox injections and Baclofen. To relieve Alice's spasticity they tried several different medications. Some just made her too groggy and irritable even though they relaxed her, but for a while the oral Baclofen was a help. It enabled her to relax just enough to move her upper body to do some basic tasks like pushing switches or reaching to choose a toy or to bicycle her legs. They visited a clinic at Children's Hospital called the Spasticity Clinic for help with this. Early on, they had decided that they would not have Alice try an experimental procedure but, if something was established and had a reasonable track record, they would. The Baclofen Pump was inserted into the abdomen just above the hip bone under the skin. A tube went from the pump around to the spine and was inserted into the spinal cord so that Baclofen could be delivered directly into the nervous system. Before the pump was inserted, a test was run where a dose of Baclofen was injected into the spine and then the response was evaluated. Alice had this procedure done in the hospital.

During her evaluation she did experience lower muscle tone and easier movement. It was much easier to take care of the basics such as getting her dressed; changing her diapers and stretching her. Two unsettling events happened, though. The first occurred while Alice was in the Children's hospital for the day. Her medicines had to be given by the hospital staff. She had been getting small doses of atropine which would dry up her saliva for a while so she did not drool as much. The doctor miscalculated the amount of drug, or wrote the dose to be administered incorrectly so when the nurse arrived in the room to give Alice her dose, Carol looked at the syringe and said that it appeared to be a lot more than she was usually given. At first the nurse said this is what the doctor ordered. Carol pulled out the syringe she usually used for comparison to the nurse's dose. It was obvious their dose was incorrect and the nurse had to get it fixed and ordered correctly. Had Carol not noticed the difference Alice would've gotten too much atropine which could have had a very detrimental result. The second issue was that Carol sent Alice to school the next day. The Andersons were never told that she should be kept still because of the needle in her spine. She ended up getting very sick at school, throwing up and having a major headache which Carol found afterwards was also a possible complication. At home, Alice was fine as long as she was lying down, but if she sat up, she seemed to get ill for a day or two afterwards. The Andersons felt badly about sending Alice to school, maintaining that no one had told them.

The results of the test were mostly positive, however. Memories of the surgery included how upset Alice was when she left her parents to go into surgery. She was so, so upset and scared despite explanations ahead of time about what was going to happen. Several weeks had been spent reading pre-school and elementary school-age books to her about being in the hospital for surgery such as "Curious George Goes to the Hospital" and a Sesame Street book. But with a non-verbal child it was hard to know how much she really understood. During the surgery, the Andersons sat in the waiting room with other parents, some of whose kids were very, very ill. When Alice's surgery was done they were told everything went well. Shortly after that a nurse came to get Carol. She couldn't tell if Alice was in pain because she couldn't talk and wanted her mother to come to the recovery room because Alice was crying. Carol went in and it was so upsetting because she was crying in a way Carol had never heard. It was almost a keening low moan over and over again. And when she saw Carol, she just did more of it, louder. Carol told the nurse, yes—she was in pain, and couldn't believe it when they told her they hadn't given Alice any pain medication yet! One would think with a child they would just assume they would need some pain medication. As soon as they did and it started to take effect, the moaning and keening sound stopped. Carol basically lived at Children's hospital for the next several days. It was a challenge to keep Alice occupied in the hospital. After speaking with the child life department, a VCR was delivered to Alice's room so she watched lots of video's as well as reading a lot of books. They also listened to Alice's favorite musical tapes including Raffi, one of her favorites. Greg was in the hospital frequently to spell Carol. Alice had trouble sleeping so Carol ended up getting into the bed with her and the two of them would sleep. It actually worked pretty well because Alice was comforted and her mother at least was in a bed instead of chair to sleep.

There were two things Carol remembered after the surgery. The first was the attempt at hydrating Alice by IV because it was difficult getting her to drink and eat in her bed. Sitting in her wheelchair at first was pretty uncomfortable. But she was so hydrated that she was urinating copiously and her diapers couldn't seem to keep up so there were many sheet changes. The other was that she did not move her legs at all. It was almost as if she was paralyzed. The doctors assured her parents that she was not. But, after having Alice usually so active with her legs kicking when she lay down, it was very worrisome. After a few days, she started some in-hospital physical therapy. One of the physical therapists gave Carol an explanation. She suggested that Alice might be afraid to move her legs because she was afraid it would hurt if she did. Eventually, movement did come back.

Alice was released home where she recovered for several weeks before going back to school. During that time, her teacher, Mary, made "home school" 'visits to the house to keep Alice's skills up. Alice's initial amount of Baclofen being administered in the pump was small but it was easier to get her dressed, or change her diaper. But the decreased muscle tone meant that in some instances Alice had to relearn how to coordinate muscle movement. For example, she had been using her thigh muscle tone to support her body weight while standing with help and walking. When her parents tried to have her stand with help and move her legs forward she just seemed to collapse. Also, feeding and giving her something to drink was initially harder. Alice went to the neurology clinic to have her pump refilled and to increase the flow rate of the Baclofen. Initially, her doses were upped by a higher rate, but the Andersons found that each time the dose was increased, Alice would go thru an adjustment period all over again. After dealing with this a few times, Carol discussed the problem with the nurse practitioner who was seen for the refills and dose increases. Smaller increases seemed to help—the more gradual changes gave Alice a chance to adjust more easily which made it easier for her parents since she would not get as frustrated. She also seemed to sleep a bit better. She was often awake at night, but not as frequently and she seemed to fall asleep and go back to sleep more easily.

While ITP therapy did help to decrease Alice's tone after her surgery, other problems arose. Alice had been using her high tone to hold up her head and keep her trunk erect. Without the high tone, she suddenly had difficulty doing these two things. She had to relearn to use her muscles to perform these tasks. With the Baclofen pump, each time it is refilled the rate that the medicine is being pumped is increased, usually by 10% each visit. Alice's adaptation to the pump decreased dramatically with each refilling, extending even to coordinating swallowing liquids including her own saliva. A rate of 5% increase in pump rate at every refill visit somewhat alleviated this problem.

Alice always had a very strong startle reflex. Usually babies outgrow this reflex, but Alice never did. Her startle reaction seemed to become less severe. Of course, the startle reflex now that Alice was older usually made her laugh at herself. The most positive change was in her upper body tone. The doctor had inserted the tubing as high as possible into her spine so as to relieve upper body tone. She was much more relaxed and able to move her arms, especially her left arm. This led eventually to greater use of augmented communication and the possibility of a self-propelled wheelchair.

Seizures

There was one large negative result from the Baclofen pump. Alice had not had any seizures since the early ones when she was first born. Baclofen can lower the seizure threshold and Carol noticed that Alice seemed to have a vacant stare shortly after her surgery. At first Carol thought it was just from being in pain or from the new sensations of having the pump. But when Alice went back to school, her summer school teacher noticed the staring and told us she thought Alice might be having petit mal seizures.

ITB therapy also decreases the point at which seizures can begin to develop because of the therapy. So, while Alice had been seizure-free since her problems at birth, she started having seizures again. These were controlled with Carbatrol, but careful monitoring of her medications was always necessary.

Alice had been followed by a neurologist yearly for a few issues such as her small head size and the possibility of seizures. After the staring episodes, testing was done to determine what type of seizures she was having. These tests were extremely challenging for Alice and her parents. They weren't painful—just impossible to do with a child as involved as Alice. The neurologist wanted to do a two hour sleep study. Alice was supposed to be kept up all night so she would be tired for the mid-morning study and fall asleep. Carol could not keep her up all night. She ended up sleeping a couple of hours. But even if she had stayed up all night there was no way she was going to fall asleep at the sleep study. Many leads were hooked up to her head and then Carol was supposed to get her to sleep. It could not be done. Alice just would not sleep and just kept on crying and trying to take the leads out of her hair. Carol calmed her down by reading to her or singing, but that would just keep her awake. Apparently not understanding, the technicians yelled at Carol for not being able to get her to sleep. Apparently, they did catch some irregular activity during the two hours Alice was wide awake. When Alice got to the neurologist later, the doctor took pity on her and decided to just treat Alice for the staring episodes based on the irregular brain activity that had been observed, and see if any other seizures happened. It seemed to him it would be almost impossible and incredibly frustrating to try to do an overnight study. The negative of not having a firm diagnosis of types of Alice's seizures was that her parents did not know if she was having any major seizures while sleeping. No one ever observed any seizures other than the staring episodes during the day. So, Alice was given a small dose of seizure medication which helped immensely in controlling the staring episodes.

Alice had initially been eating baby food longer than most kids would. During preschool the teachers, speech and occupational therapists tried to teach Alice to chew and drink from a cup. It was quickly discovered after a visit to the Swallowing Clinic that Alice had a swallowing disorder and all of her liquids needed to be thickened since otherwise she would choke. She was still using a bottle and it took many years for her to learn to use a cup well enough to totally give up her bottle. Her liquids were supplemented by giving her a bottle in the afternoon after school and before bed. She never learned how to chew, so, for her whole life food was ground up. Dinner, for example, was what the family was eating ground up, with ice cream for dessert. And Alice LOVED ice cream. When she was older she also loved chocolate sundaes with whipped cream. The biggest challenge was eating out. The Andersons would either have to bring ground up food previously heated and put in a thermos or use a fork to finely mush up either spaghetti or mac 'n cheese. Eventually they used a battery operated grinder that was portable to grind up restaurant food. It was always a production. Pre-checking a restaurant's menu to make sure there was something Alice could eat, then, when the meal was served, grinding up the food. Of course, one of her parents had to feed Alice and usually their food would get cold. As soon as one parent was done eating, the other would take over feeding Alice so the first could eat. Before Alice used a wheelchair, a special booster chair was obtained, after trying many models, which was portable and could be attached to restaurant chairs. Pillows were used to prop Alice correctly.

At home, usually Carol fed Alice breakfast and a snack after school and Greg would feed her dinner. Feeding Alice especially when she was younger was quite the challenge and very frustrating. She had a very strong tongue thrust that took a very long time to stop her from doing. Half of the food put in her mouth would immediately come back out. If she was very tired, it would be even worse. And if either Greg or Carol were tired they would lose patience. They knew it wasn't Alice's fault, but it required a lot of talking to her and special techniques to feed her, even with a specialized spoon. The therapist and teachers at school were a huge help in teaching her parents how to work through these issues, but none of it was learned quickly by Alice or, for that matter, her parents. It would take many years to perfect the simplest things. She was constantly told her keep her tongue in her mouth. She would thrust her tongue out all the time, even when she wasn't eating. Again, someone touched her tongue when she did it and say "tongue in". Eventually she learned to keep her tongue in her mouth. She even learned to indicate she was thirsty by doing tongue thrusts voluntarily.

While still in her first house, Alice got her first wheelchair. The house was not wheelchair accessible. To get Alice into or out of the house the wheelchair had to be tilted back and dragged up or down three steps. Her bedroom was on the first floor luckily, but the hallways and bathroom were narrow. During Alice's early years, she was in a special program which provided government financial help to families with special needs children. The program only looked at Alice's income, which was negligible and was based on the premise that children such as she would probably be institutionalized. The support was cheaper if they remained at home with their families. The financial help included diapers, secondary insurance, equipment and home modifications. A ramp was built onto the back of the house to provide accessibility. Unfortunately there was no way to modify the bathroom in the house at the time.

Over and over, people characterized Alice as a happy child. Her smile would brighten their days and her laughter seemed to reflect the joy and love in her heart. She was happiest when experiencing life to its fullest and the Andersons tried to support that. Alice loved roller coasters so they traveled to amusement parks where Greg would hold onto her for dear life on the more sane rides. That way she could experience the thrill she loved. She loved taking her dog for a walk on her adaptive tricycle. Carol pushed Alice and her bike around the neighborhood. They wanted her to be happy, and from the statements people made, she truly was a happy child which showed as she went about her daily activities. The late actor Christopher Reeve once said, to paraphrase, "A functional family when faced with adversity draws strength from each other and becomes closer—a dysfunctional family when faced with difficulties falters and is torn apart." The Andersons were happy and strong. They still are. Both Carol and Greg were family oriented to begin with. Both are physically fit and strong. The family's endurance throughout Alice's life and subsequent events would be proof of that.

Alice's favorite TV personality was Barney. She would watch him for hours, and laugh. Often, early on, her brother, G3, would watch with her sometimes with both their heads propped up on Disco their dog. Barney's unique purple color became a large part of Alice's wardrobe.

That is not to say that it was easy to take care of Alice—everything required more time, effort and energy. But then, their philosophy was, the best things in life always required more work. Life with a child with a disability might seem difficult or an extra burden or even inconvenient to many, but for the Andersons, that was just the way it was and they were accepting of it. It was just life with the daughter they loved. And even though she couldn't talk, or walk or even feed herself, she gave much back to them with her love, spirit and positive attitude despite her disabilities.

When Alice was at home after her birth, it became obvious to one and all that Greg and Carol were sleep deprived. This was, in part, because both parents were intent upon maintaining their normal schedules, such as Greg's running five miles every morning, very early, despite the weather. Both of Alice's parents naturally approach life with great determination and intensity. But mainly, as Grammy still puts it, "Alice never slept." Truly, she had what everyone came to call "power naps", which was fine during the day, but was not the best sleeping habit at night. Alice had a strong startle response and would frequently startle herself awake at night. She couldn't switch her position in her bed at night so she would often wake up briefly and she would have to be rolled over to her other side. The Andersons took turns going to her, alternating so that each of them could get some sleep. They remained chronically sleep-deprived and so anything that would help Alice to sleep a little better was to be sought after. Every once in a blue moon, Alice would sleep all night long and that was a blessing, except that then Alice's mother and father would fear that something was wrong with her.

Of course, there were the usual things one had to do for a newborn, not the least of which was food preparation. And Carol continued to pump her breast to feed her daughter for several months. So this took twice as long as normal breast feeding. Alice never could learn how to breast feed. It was just too hard for her to learn to coordinate efficiently enough to do so, although Carol really did try to teach her. Much of that was done in the evening before bedtime. After a feeding, when most babies would go back to sleep, Alice did not. Hence, one or the other of her parents was awake during the night. In the early years, Alice's grandparents would wonder if Greg and Carol ever had a full night's sleep. So, she was a terrible sleeper. She never napped more than 10 to 20 minutes and rarely slept through the night perhaps because she could not turn over.

Almost from the time she came home from the hospital, Alice underwent physical therapy. This was administered by her parents, often first thing in the morning and at other times during the day. These were mainly passive stretching exercises. Since Alice was not a "morning person" she was usually not happy about this, but the exercises were not painful to her. Carol is a personal trainer, so this kind of therapy for Alice came naturally to her mother. (Carol, it is noted again here, had planned to stay at work after she gave birth, but in the end had to give up her promising career in the insurance industry. Greg continued his work at an international engineering organization in The City.)

Just as she had taken her own breast milk to the hospital each day, Carol continued to feed Alice breast milk at home.

Alice had early intervention at home. Physical therapy, stretching exercises. People came to the house at first and then "Allie", as she came to be called, was taken elsewhere for her therapy. She was to have stretching and exercises each day for the rest of her life.

And Alice was difficult to feed. Swallowing was a problem for her. She needed to have all her liquids thickened with a product called "Thick-it" to a consistency of very thick honey. Eventually, she had been having more problems with her swallowing. She seemed to be choking on her own saliva. Dr. Anderson, Alice's grandfather, commented on this when she was visiting Florida. While there, she had problems while eating—gasping for breath almost as if she were choking. Her teacher and speech therapist as well as her baby sitter also noted this to Carol. She did control some of her life by her reaction to being fed. If she was unhappy about something, she would make feeding her even more difficult than it already was. People who cared for her were able eventually to figure out the meaning of some of this communication.

Alice also had a history of recurrent sinus infections, often in the spring. Hence, because of nasal congestion, the head of her bed was slightly elevated to help her breathe more easily. She was unable to blow her nose. If she got a cold it invariably would lead to a sinus infection. Just a cold would mean she would have even more trouble sleeping. A humidifier was used in her room as well as a saline nasal spray with limited success. The head end of her specialty bed was raised to help her breathe. If she needed medicine, whether it was just a decongestant, liquid Motrin, or an antibiotic it was quite a challenge. Alice almost always spit it out. Pills didn't work because she choked on them. Crushing up the pills and hiding them in her food didn't work because she could taste the difference and just wouldn't eat the food. She just wouldn't swallow it. In the end the only thing that for the most part worked was to put small amounts of liquid medicine in her mouth while she was lying down and getting her to swallow it somehow. Tylenol suppositories were used for fever because that was just much simpler to do.

Alice also had quite severe chronic constipation. Normally, a suppository that stimulated a bowel movement was used. She would receive enemas several times a week. At one point, a doctor had her parents making milk and molasses enemas—warming milk and melting molasses in it. That became too much to handle with everything else the Andersons had to do.

When Alice was little, Grammy Millie was able to help out with her by making items for her with all sorts of uses. There were foam rubber pillows, wedges for her bed and other items to help support her as well as sleep mats which Alice could use while lying on the floor. She often used fabrics with fanciful prints. Many of these items ended up with names such as a roll to help support Alice covered in a print featuring hippotamuses, the famous "hippo roll".

Millie also made dresses for Alice. Alice's dresses had to be constructed so that they were more easily used in the wheel chair. A quilted robe, for instance, was made shorter in the back so it would be easier to put Alice into and out of the chair but the robe could still be tied around her.

Grammy also does prize-winning smocking and she would make matching smocked dresses for her two granddaughters. One time, a friend asked her in all seriousness, why Millie would even make such a dress for Alice, too. Aghast, Millie replied, "Why not? Allie is just as much my granddaughter as Meghan (the Anderson's oldest granddaughter)."

Alice was always beautifully dressed, always in age and activity-appropriate clothes. Unfortunately, her drooling was non-stop since she could not swallow her saliva correctly. Carol's solution was to use easily laundered "bandannas" which were tied loosely around her neck and always "went with" her outfit. In the end, Alice had a huge number of scarves, which eventually found other uses.

The summer after Alice, by now frequently called Allie, was born, the family came to visit the Andersons. There was a lovely pool at their house with a cabana just off the family room. Greg and Carol seemed to be doing very well, but were very stressed out as was everyone. They were snapping at each other until Millie, despite living by the motto "ears open, mouth closed" decided on a slight intervention.

She called Greg into the cabana and announced that we were all very concerned and that they, Greg and Carol, were not going to make if they kept up with the short tempers and the snapping at each other. (Greg could be overly critical at times and Carol was all set sometimes to have things her way.) Millie felt strongly that they had to work as a team to be able to keep on dealing with Allie successfully. From that time until this day Millie is so thankful that "the kids" got their act together. She didn't think that they would make it through, even when the future difficulties were unknown, if they weren't together as a team.

Alice loved to go for walks, first in her stroller and later in her wheel chair. Once, when G3 was born and Grammy was in Maneta to help, she took Allie for "walks" in the neighborhood. She would get her numerous propping pillows arranged in the stroller and off they would go. As much as Millie thought that she had her emotions under control, they would surface when she would see perfectly normal kids playing outdoors and this child and her parents would never see this with Alice. Those emotions surfaced numerous times over the years. Even now many years later, they occasionally do.

Eventually, Alice began to have regular school-type classes. Alice's bus would pick her up at 7:00 am and return her to her house at 4:30 pm. This seemed like a longer interval away from home than would be expected for a normal student. So, one day, Alice's father followed the bus. It turned out that she had a two hour ride each way from school. The Andersons contacted the school transportation department which refused to do anything about the length of the ride. Another parent of a child with a disability indicated that Carol should get a note indicating that, medically, Alice couldn't be on the bus longer than an hour. When Carol contacted Alice's pediatrician, he was more than happy to help. From then on Alice practically had limousine service to and from school!

The Andersons eventually purchased a green high-top conversion van. It was a great vehicle as it enabled video games for G3, videos for Alice. This, of course, was before having a video screen in one's vehicle was common. The elder Andersons initially thought that a minivan would be an improvement over taking apart Alice's wheelchair and putting the pieces of it in their car trunk in order for them to go anywhere. The minivan did allow Carol and Greg to put just the chair in the back of the van. The repeated lifting of the chair however, was giving Carol major back problems. So, as a result of the lawsuit they were able to buy the bigger van. At the time, it was quite the luxury. The vehicle also had two separate sound systems so the driver and front seat passenger could actually listen to music while the kids in the back watched a video. There was a very special lift into the van where Alice's wheelchair would attach by strong straps to an arm that would swing her into the vehicle. Then she would be rolled over to her spot and the floor anchors attached to her wheelchair. This way there was not a large lift covering the side doorway. The van worked out very well and made it very comfortable in which to take road trips. The vanity plate read "ALICEBUS". The van is gone now, but the license plate remains in use. The family was able to take many vacations to fun places like Cedar Point Amusement Center, Myrtle Beach, Florida, Hershey Park in PA as well as trips to see family.

One problem, though, was that the high top of the van made a few things challenging. For example, when Carol had to take Alice to Children's Hospital for an appointment, which was often, she couldn't park the van in the parking garage—it was too tall. Trying to find parking on the street with a large van is not easy. So, eventually a second vehicle, a smaller van which had an automatic ramp in it was purchased. The ramp was super convenient and having two vehicles with the capability to take Alice in them was wonderful. All of this specialized equipment would not have been possible if not for the settlement from Alice's lawsuit and it really improved the quality of life for the whole family.

Plane rides were a different matter. Of course, the Anderson's pre-boarded; while Carol kept an eye on the wheel chair, Greg had to carry Alice to her seat. At first they tried using a car seat on the plane, but that did not work out. Eventually, Alice would be strapped into her seat surrounded by pillows for support.

At destination, the boarding procedure would be repeated in reverse. An Anderson cousin, spoken of in Greg's pretrial testimony, told them about a magazine entitled "Exceptional Parent". It was from this publication that the Andersons learned about rental "Wheelchair Getaways". This firm would pick the Andersons up at the airport and deliver them to their destination. They were then able to use the special van provided by

Wheelchair Getaways until they were picked up once again and taken to the airport for the trip home. This arrangement was exceedingly helpful for all and greatly increased everyone's ability to relax while on vacation.

Alice was also very busy with her "adaptive" sport and recreational activities. These included:

Horseback riding: Alice attended a Therapeutic Riding Center, at a horseback riding stable nearby. This was an accredited therapeutic riding center recognized by the North American Riding for the Handicapped Association. Horseback riding was provided to riders challenged by physical, mental or emotional disabilities. During the time the trainer was director of the Center, she worked with Alice thirty-two weeks out of the year for five years. As such, she was very familiar with Alice's physical abilities and disabilities as they made themselves obvious in the program.

Several reasons were important in the decision to have Alice do horseback riding. It was an activity Alice could do on weekends during the summer with the goal being to have some fun and possibly to help with her nighttime sleeping. Therapeutic riding had been shown to assist people with disabilities in their trunk control and the movement of the horse simulated what it was like to walk. Also, the warmth and the movement of the horse were supposed to help decrease muscle tone and aid in hip flexibility.

Alice especially liked to canter, of course, because it was faster and bumpy. It always made her laugh. Carol also noticed a difference in Alice's flexibility as the summer went on—looser hips and hamstrings. Holding her head and torso erect seemed also to improve.

Because of her physical disabilities, Alice was unable to ride without considerable assistance and support. Specifically, Alice did not have the ability to hold her torso or head up for any length of time. Thus, in order for Alice to ride, she was provided with a special vest. The vest was secured around her torso. There were two straps, one on either side of the vest near waist level and two handles near the top of the vest at the shoulders.

Whenever Alice rode a horse, she was accompanied on either side by two "sidewalkers" who were employees of the Center. Each of the sidewalkers placed one arm through the vest straps at Alice's waist and held the handles at the top of the vest. Thus, they were completely supporting Alice's torso and keeping her erect. All riders rode on a blanket with a steel bar in front of them so that they could hold onto the bar as they rode. When Alice rode, this bar was wrapped with padding because she was unable to hold up her torso or her head if the side walkers lost control of her. She was the only rider with this protection

The Director of the center noted that a photograph of Alice riding might be interpreted as showing that Alice had some ability to control her head and neck. As someone who worked extensively with Alice, the Director was able to state that Alice had only limited and weak control of her head and could maintain this control for only very brief periods of time. Unfortunately, after the Baclofen pump was implanted, she had to relearn torso and head control.

At a later date, the Riding Center planted a tree in Alice's honor complete with a plaque.

Ice skating: Alice and her whole family were deeply involved with an ice skating program available locally. At first, Alice's parents were, at least in part, looking for an activity to do with Alice on weekends which would get her moving and perhaps tire her out a bit so that she might sleep deeper at night. Getting Alice to sleep longer at night was always a goal. There were also stories of children who had made tremendous strides physically when they started skating. There were miracle stories of kids who had been unable to walk, and who became able to do so because of their skating programs. Since the Andersons were still trying to learn to "accept" Alice's disabilities, these stories definitely appealed to them.

Alice went weekly to the skating venue in The City, the professional hockey team players' ice arena, from October through March. Over 600 skaters from near and far came to the program. Parents and caregivers were involved with all the children as well volunteers, often high school students, who donated untold hours teaching the sport to disabled children. Many of the children, such as Alice, required specialized equipment in order to participate. Many did not and some made phenomenal advances in their athletic ice skating abilities. To this end, Alice's parents and her brother instituted the Alice Anderson Spirit Award, still given annually to a skater who has made a "spirited" effort to improve his or her ice skating.

The family arrived at the skating venue the first day with Alice in her hot pink wheelchair. G3 was a toddler and Alice was still at the point where she would scream bloody murder if Carol walked a few feet away from her. The first day of the season was always reserved for getting fitted for skates with limited time on the ice. Skates were specially designed to accommodate all the different needs of the skater. This first day was a difficult one for all. Since a harness would not work for her, a sling seat was suggested for her. It was decided that Carol would try being one of the volunteers for Alice, hoping that would calm her down. Carol had had experience as an ice skater during her childhood and teens. Indeed, the first season was not an easy one for Alice since she did not like the slow parts of practice—she loved the fast parts. However, Alice eventually got to the point where she could last at least an hour. Eventually, one of Alice's volunteers was a young man who had been a star of the program and had progressed enough to become a volunteer.

Each year there is a "Celebration on Ice" show at the arena. Alice's grandparents and other family members were privileged several times to see this program. It was hard to imagine the colorful and complicated routines that these children with their helpers were able to perform. The show costumes were all made by volunteers. One act consisted of 500 Winnie-the-Poohs filling the arena ice. Alice's first show was memorable and Carol felt quite emotional about it. Going out on the ice with the arena crowd cheering the skaters was a moment Carol had never believed would happen when Alice was born. It was transforming in that it helped the Andersons understand that Alice would have her own accomplishments and could be helped to become the best she could be. While that "best" was different from a typical kid, it was still the goal that any parent would want for their child.

A professional, sometimes an Olympic ice skating star, also contributed time to the program.

Over the years, Alice continued to progress. The big moment came when, one season, she started to "bicycle" her feet and to use the teeth part of the skate blade to dig into the ice and then to move herself forward. Eventually she could propel herself half way around the rink.

The Andersons continued to make improvements in Alice's equipment. Important was the use of walkers. These gave Alice much more support through her torso, helping her to move her feet more. They also helped her to bear weight which was so important for her bone growth and health. So, skating became medically important fun for Alice. Eventually, not unexpectedly, with Alice at over five feet tall and weighing 120 pounds, getting her onto the ice with all her equipment became very hard work.

Greg and Carol were used to making all of Alice's activities as therapeutic as possible because it was important for them to use all opportunities to help Alice make strides in overcoming her physical and mental disabilities.

Dance: Alice's dance program was one which she especially enjoyed and seemed also to benefit from. The Andersons had learned early on that music and movement brought a smile to Alice's face and helped to calm her. Even as a baby, the only way they could get her to nap was to put her into the swing and let the movement induce her to sleep. According to a description of the dance program, sessions were provided in a safe, non-threatening environment for individuals to grow and develop to their own potentials. Instruction focused on the essentials of movement, expanding each individual's natural kinesthetic repertoire and studying a dance style in modified or technical form. The Moving Miracles organization's premise stems from an holistic approach which encourages the mind/body connection. Dance/movement is explored using one's body and a variety of props, musical selections and tools such as visualization, imaging and mirroring. The experience also includes spacial relations, sensory integration, body awareness and concept formation in relation to one's own and other's environment. Tuition was required.

Life experiences, which most of us take for granted, are vital and intrinsic to the continued development of each student's mental, physical and emotional potential.

Alice came to her dance program the first year, her parent's knowing that movement and music could help, but totally unsure as to how director, Ms. S., was going to get Alice to "dance". Alice was one of the program's first students. Alice and Carol were impressed from the beginning. Ms. S. and her volunteers used the most creative ways to coax movement out of Alice who just squealed in delight at being able to move any way she wanted while having fun. During the first year, Carol agreed to serve on the newly created Board of Directors while helping the program to attain non-profit status.

In Alice's class, the students were paired with a volunteer who would use hand over hand or hand over another part of her body to assist her in movement. Volunteers were high school dance students doing community service. Later, the program had college students studying special education, physical occupation and speech therapy as well as dancers. The very first year, the program ended with a recital.

Alice thrived in the environment at the studio, making friends and learning to move using her own movement patterns which led to accomplishments in therapy and at school. Because the students in Alice's class were so physically involved, the recitals usually were choreographed pieces that had Alice in a wheelchair partnering with her volunteer dancing. The students would wear beautiful costumes but the volunteers always dressed in black—they were shadows assisting the dancers.

The classes themselves involved movement on mats or while the students sat in the volunteers' laps, wearing tap-dancing shoes while the volunteers assisted in the tapping of the students' feet. Just the sound of feedback of their feet in tap shoes helped students try to move to make the sounds.

Dance class was a program that gave parents a break as well. While Alice was in class, Carol would sit in the waiting area chatting with the other moms. A lot of emotional support, therapy ideas, and brainstorming of problems were done during the hour the group waited for their children.

Carol was often mistress of ceremonies for the recital. Nowadays, volunteering for the program has become a way for the Andersons to honor their daughter and sister as they saw her joy in life that the spotlight highlighted on stage. For the annual recital the family works backstage or operates the lights. Several of G3's friends also help while his high school National Honor Society group has become involved in volunteering.

Recently, one young man was to go on stage, but, unfortunately, the anxiety, nervousness and stress of waiting to perform were getting to him and he was having a "meltdown". After quickly juggling the order of the program, the volunteers were able to get him on stage for his solo. The music played and the spotlight shined as he tapped out his routine. When he took his bows to thunderous applause, the smile on his face was the most amazing thing to see. His accomplishment was a triumph. As he came off the stage, he excitedly said to his teacher, "I was great. I did it!" Carol watched his Mom crying tears of joy when she came backstage and Carol knew how she felt. Carol had felt that way at Alice's first performance years before. Carol noted that, "When you have a child with a disability, you never imagine you will ever get a chance to watch your kid get applause on a stage in the spotlight. While your friends are taking their kids to ballet class or karate class, you are worrying about your child's speech therapy or what goals you should push for in her Educational Plan or if your insurance appeal for equipment will be approved". Moments of accomplishment such as this help in the healing process as parents move toward acceptance and peace with their child with a disability.

Swimming: Alice loved the water. This included getting wet on an amusement park water ride and especially in the pool. There were always people to see to her safety. Millie could only hold her and participate when Alice was in the pool. Foam rubber "noodles" and inner tubes were used to support her and to guide her while she cavorted in the pool. The more she got splashed, the better she liked it! Being in the water was one of Alice's favorite activities. She responded to it well and was able to be herself in something that was different from her everyday world. Not a wheelchair, not a walker, just, to her, good-old-everyday fun out of her everyday routine. Although a lot of work for her parents, they made every effort to get her to the pool and into the water. Possibly, she was the example that G3 followed in pursuing a swimming career in high school.

The first time Alice went swimming she was not overly fond of it. She cried her typical reaction to new things when she was little. It wasn't until Greg began to goof around with her after one or two times that she became a fan of the water.

Alice had been started in Red Cross swim lessons when she was an infant and toddler. Eventually she aged out of the lessons technically, but, of course, skill-wise she had not aged out of the infant/toddler skills. After that, Carol took Alice to a local pool when there was time. This was another way for her to have some therapeutic care as well as to tire her out. After Alice had a Baclofen Pump placed, swimming became a bit more complicated. However, she began water therapy at a local physiotherapy office. The nearness of the office to home and the warmed water also helped.

A physiatrist noted that Alice's bone density was excellent and felt that the many physical activities in which Alice participated were the reason. On the doctor's recommendation, the Andersons were able to install an in-ground pool at their home which was tax-deductible.

Adaptive Skiing: While making sure G3 learned to ski, the Andersons heard about adaptive ski programs in their area, one of which could handle a multi-handicapped student. Alice enjoyed her time with the expert skiers who volunteered in the program and she loved to go downhill fast, of course.

Alice would use a "sit-ski" which meant she sat on a seat, strapped in, which was on a broad double ski which was fairly stable. If Alice leaned over too much, it would tip over. Alice never minded being tipped over in the snow and sometimes it made her laugh. A very strong skier would be holding onto a harness that was attached to the sit-ski. The skier would be behind Alice helping to steer or slow her down. Another expert skier would actually ski in front of her trying to get her to lean slightly and turn the ski herself. A third skier followed directing others away from the group as they skied by. Alice also got to ride the chairlift since her seat could be lifted up, placed on the ski lift chair which was locked into place. Two skiers sat on either side of her. The whole procedure was ingenious, rather incredible. While Alice was having her lesson which lasted two hours, the rest of the family would ski. Then came lunch, after which someone would stay to entertain Alice while the others continued to ski. It became a fun way to pass a winter's day while enjoying a normal activity.

Skiing was a wonderful thing for Alice since it was something totally different from what she was used to. She was away from her parents and brother and was able to challenge herself to the capacity she knew she had. She had to rely on her assistants to have a successful day. Skiing also allowed Alice to experience things on her own. She never really got too upset getting ready to ski . . . . maybe she knew her instructors were going to make things fast and exciting.

T-ball: Here, the ball is large and soft. Able-bodied aids were present to help Alice participate, such has moving her wheelchair around the bases. Some organizations have rules which were it not for the handicaps in evidence, would be amusing. All participants play each inning, everyone is always safe at base, each team wins every game and the like. An objective such as improved hand-eye coordination is important.

This was one of Alice's activities that got her involved and out in the community. It was evident, however, that she would much rather be roaming the bases than playing second base! Too sedentary for her to be hanging out in the field. Also, the game was played on a normal baseball field, dirt, grass and all. The part Alice liked was getting bumped while she was pushed around the bases.

Alice also had a tricycle and a talking computer. The computer was used to help her communicate to pick an afterschool activity. She could pick reading books, music to listen to or a game to play. If the weather was nice, she could indicate the swing in the backyard or her tricycle. If Alice was being pushed on her tricycle, the Anderson's dog, Disco always came along.

At Halloween, Alice always had wonderful costumes. Once she was Cinderella in a costume which Grammy made for her. She had poster board pumpkins as windows on her wheelchair, a prize-winning outfit. Alice was Pocahontas, the Energizer Bunny and GI Jane, among other characters.

Chapter 5

Schooling

Alice would age into the preschool therapy program right around her second birthday. This level involved a school based program with a teacher and aides working with a small group of students with similar issues. Alice's therapies would be one-on-one and occur during the day at school. A bus would pick her up in the morning and bring her home in the mid-afternoon. When Carol was pregnant with Alice, she would imagine her life and various milestones—she never imagined the first day of school would be handing her two year old off to a bus monitor to have her buckled into a car seat on the bus, waving goodbye and praying the monitor had buckled her in properly.

Alice actually started the preschool program in the winter before G3 was born. She was started initially for a half day so she could get used to going to school. Carol went to get her right after lunch. Carol remembers thinking that starting the program early was good because Alice would be used to it by the time the baby arrived and would not associate suddenly going away to school with the birth of her brother. Having her in school would also give Carol more time to spend with the baby for a while which would be helpful since Alice's care was still that of an infant. It would be like having twins in many ways.

The special education infant and preschool programs included a six week summer session as well. Alice continued her program through the summer. Carol still picked her up after lunch but, starting in September after G3 was born, Alice began to stay the full day. Her first teacher was Mrs. Kirk who had been a special education teacher for many years and was wonderful. Alice was in a class of highly involved pre-school kids with similar issues who required a lot of one-on-one assistance. Mrs. Kirk had three aides in the classroom to assist her. In many ways the class was like any preschool. There was circle time where "learning songs" were sung, playtime where the teacher and aides worked with the preschoolers on their individual goals, crafts, snack time, lunch, quiet or nap-time, etc. The students would also get their physical, occupational and speech therapies, usually in a separate therapy room. There were also gym, art and music teachers who would work with the classes once or twice a week. The students even went on field trips such as to the zoo or the farm.

It was during preschool that the tradition of Alice's notebook started. The teachers would send home a notebook in her backpack every day with a note telling her parents how Alice's day had been, what they had done that day and whether Alice had had a good day. The Andersons always returned a nice note to the teacher telling them what Alice had done after school or over the weekend so the teacher would have something to talk to Alice about. They also would tell the teacher what Alice's lunch was. The school did have lunch to buy and, on occasion if there was something Alice liked which would grind up well, they would send in money. For the most part, however, they would send in a ground up meal for the staff to heat up. Enough food for dinner was cooked so that Alice's lunch for the next day was provided for. And she ate well. That was partly why she never was so skinny and as frail looking as so many of her friends at school. Over the years the teachers loved her healthy, hearty meals—although the fish might have caused a few "odor" issues when it was heated up. Her parents would mix some low sodium, low fat gravy into ground up steak, or BBQ sauce into the chicken breast, add a little water and butter to veggies and grind them up. Even rice and noodles could be made palatable. Then they would send in ground up canned fruit for dessert or occasionally send in money for ice cream. Her juice or milk had to be sent in thickened as well—they went through many, many yellow cans of "Thick-it".

Alice's progress at school was evaluated carefully. The teacher and therapists would set up individual goals for her along with parental input. The goals were simple, i.e.: Alice was to reach out and push a big red switch to activate a toy when prompted, 3 out of 5 tries. She was to hold onto a rattle toy and shake it 2 out of 5 attempts. The goals would then be grouped together into an individual education plan (IEP) and would be submitted to the school district Committee on Preschool Special Education along with the teachers' and therapists' recommendations on the number of times per week the therapy should take place. The parents, teachers and Committee would then review the IEP and, hopefully, accept it. Goals could be changed or updated during the course of the year. From the very first meeting, Carol and Greg made it a point to attend the Committee meetings. Also included in the IEP were any equipment needs to be used at school. If the child needed the equipment to be educated in the State, the school district would have to provide it. At grammar school age and beyond, the situation was similar except the Committee became the Committee on Special Education. Greg and Carol attended every single meeting of this committee, too.

When Alice was 5 years old, she aged out of the teaching/therapy program and she began to attend BOCES classes. Fortunately, the class she was placed in was in one of the local elementary schools. The Boards of Cooperative Educational Services (BOCES) placed classes around the State in area schools where there were empty classrooms. This was satisfactory because being in a "regular" elementary school would afford Alice opportunities for integration with her non-disabled peers. The challenge was to find the right opportunity that would allow integration to be successful for her and not a disruption for the academic classes. Many teachers were not so enthusiastic about special needs kids coming into their classrooms. The level of support given to the integration process from the building principal was another factor in how successful integration could be. Alice's new teacher was Sue West who was an experienced teacher who had worked for many years with special education students. She also had three aides assisting her. BOCES therapists would either be assigned to the schools or travel to the schools. Alice, at that point, continued to receive the maximum amount of therapy—three times a week for speech, occupational, and physical therapy. The program also provided numerous field trips into the community. A notebook was the primary means of communication with the teacher and therapists. Carol often would drop in at the classroom to check on things and would bring G3 along. After the first year, some integration was arranged during either morning circle in the kindergarten classes or when the teacher was reading books or perhaps doing a craft. But Sue West also had older kids come into the classroom to help out.

Alice stayed in this class for many years even after her family was in its new house. She did well and slowly continued to progress. She was a very happy, well-adjusted kid who seemed to enjoy school and the interactions with staff and students. Much of her learning, drawing, crafts, music etc. had to be accomplished with hand over hand help which was why the classroom had so many aides. They worked on trying to improve the daily care skills as well as academic skills of the highly involved students in the class. Carol remembers one of Alice's goals was to hold her brush and try to brush her hair. This did not work out too well because Alice was very stiff and spastic, through her upper body and arms. Another goal was holding her own spoon and feeding herself. The occupational therapist had designed a specialty spoon that was strapped with Velcro onto her hand. Alice actually often would lift up her left arm straight, then bend her elbow and put her hand into her mouth. She seemed to practice this from the time she was small and actually got very good at it. Thus, there was some limited success with her feeding herself as long as she was helped to get food on the spoon hand over hand. But it was a very cumbersome and lengthy process and ended up not being practical in most situations. As parents, the Andersons had to pick and choose what skills to focus on. Some just had to be abandoned because it wasn't going to work in the real world. She had better luck with more gross motor skills like moving a walker forward by bicycling her legs. She also was able to use her left hand to start working on an augmented communication device. Any kind of communication was a priority. Being able to communicate simple things like hunger, sickness or to choose what toy to play with became more important to her parents especially as, after a time, they realized Alice would always require one-on-one assistance. Alice's parents were quite good at understanding her and the little signs she would make to indicate what she wanted. For example, she could say "mmmm" and "gud" (good). So, she would tell them she liked a particular food by saying "mmmm gud". She was very expressive when she didn't like something—that was obvious. When she was thirsty she would repeatedly stick her tongue out as if she was going suck on a bottle. But if something hurt on her body, her parents could never tell what was wrong or hurting other than that something was wrong and she was just grumpy. If she had a temperature for more than a day, Carol would have to take her into the doctor to have her checked to make sure she didn't have an infection or pneumonia.

After Alice was in school for several years, the Andersons became aware of some issues with the classroom. The biggest one was the lack of accessibility to the second floor in the school. A ramp had been added to the front of the school so wheelchairs could access the first floor which is where the gym and auditorium were but there was not an elevator to the second floor which is where the library and some of the other special areas such as art were. So the teachers and librarian were coming to the classroom to do the projects or read books, but it meant that the wheelchair-bound students spent just about all of their time in one classroom. As Alice got older, a concern became her limited opportunities to integrate and to experience new environments and situations. In addition, there seemed to be a definite opposition to integration among the staff. They understood that placing Alice in a class that was doing math problems was inappropriate, but having her participate during art or music class was doable and Alice really enjoyed interacting with other, able kids.

The first September after the move to the new house, the bus ride became a major issue. The Anderson's new house was a 45 minute drive from the school. Alice was on the bus pretty early in the morning to get to school. Every year at the end of August the bus number and time of pick-up was mailed out. It was always an early time in the morning and Alice was not a morning person. Carol would have to get her up, stretch and do her range of motion exercises, change her diaper, get her dressed, brush her hair into a ponytail, and take her to the kitchen in her wheelchair to eat something before school. She hated getting her hair brushed when she was younger and would complain in her non-verbal way the whole time. She also was never very hungry early in the morning. So her mother basically had to try to get her to eat at least a half bowl of instant oatmeal, drink some juice and eat a little fruit so she would not be totally starving in an hour when she did finally wake up more. Some days it was a real challenge as she would just spit back the oatmeal. If Carol could wait even a half hour to feed her such as on holidays, Alice would gobble up the oatmeal so Carol knew she liked it. She just didn't want to eat that early. Her parents would try to distract her with a cartoon on TV but some days were just a struggle. If the bus was even just a couple of minutes early it meant some mornings her feeding couldn't be finished. The first set of bus drivers and aides were not at all understanding. They got angry if Alice and Carol were not out the door as soon as they showed up even if they were a minute or two early. Carol needed every minute she could get. So one year, the time the transportation department was picking Alice up was almost two hours before the start of school—just after 6 o'clock in the morning. At first Carol and Greg tried to get Alice up and meet that time, but it really was a struggle.

The last two years Alice was at this school, her teacher retired and the new teacher, Mary Tanner came into the classroom. Mary was very good and was very supportive of integration. The change for the Andersons as parents was anxiety producing, but in the end, was very good for Alice. Mary had new ideas, new crafts, and was willing to fight for some interactive integration opportunities for her students. Many of the aides in the classroom had been there for years, and there seemed to be some staff issues initially which eventually sorted themselves out. Mary Tanner helped Greg and Carol focus on goals that they would need to work towards for the time in the future when Alice became an adult, such as communication and the ability to use a self-propelled wheelchair. With Mary, what was anticipated for Alice as an adult became a focus. Mary, prior to coming to this classroom had worked with older special education students. Greg and Carol, over many conversations, developed a goal for Alice's being in a group home while they were alive perhaps with several of the friends she had made over the years in her class or at her extra activities such as skating or Moving Miracles. If a group of parents got together to purchase or build a group home, it could be run by one of the area agencies, but there would be some "checks" on the staff by several caring families. Her parents felt that to keep Alice at home would create problems down the road. What would happen when her family couldn't take care of her? She would be so used to being at home after so many years, adjustment would be very difficult. They felt that G3 would have responsibility to make sure his sister was cared for, but it was unfair, probably impossible, for him to have to take care of her day to day as her parents did. He needed to have his own life. Transitioning her to a group home when she was in her twenties where she could be visited, or come home for weekends, was important. That changed the focus of the goals for Alice as a pre-teen and teenager.

The Andersons were very excited to learn at a Committee of Special Education meeting that their new school district was going to try to keep its kids in-district by having BOCES special education classes in the schools. The town had just completed several building renovations which increased some the classroom space at the elementary school level. Alice was placed in a class at one of the elementary schools that was, at most, 15 minutes from her home. The Andersons were glad because of the new opportunities for Alice but as parents, they were very nervous about how Alice would react to the changes. Carol made sure to take Alice into the school classroom to meet the teacher ahead of time so it would not be strange for Alice. On the first day of school, the usual bus driver and aide picked her up, which probably helped her adjustment since not everything was different. She went to her new school and class without a hitch and really became one of the stars of the classroom with her happy, sunny personality. Change had been difficult for Alice in the past, but she apparently was growing up and change wasn't as scary for her now. Her new school was such a wonderful place for her. There were two special education classes in the building. Her new class was taught by Judy Cooper. Mary Tanner's class, Allie's old class and teacher, were also moved to the building. This new class was at a little higher intellectual level which was definitely more stimulating for her. And she was able to have lots of interaction with her non-disabled peers. The support of the teachers who taught special subjects like art and music was amazing. The art teacher would write notes in Alice's notebook because Alice went to an integrative art class. The teacher even showed up at a Central School Education meeting to find out how she could help Alice improve.

The people in the classroom befriended Alice and would interact with her in other situations. The whole school, including the special education classes, went to a morning program. Kids knew Alice outside of school, something that never happened back at her old class. For example, Alice, G3 and Carol would go to the library and invariably there would be a child who would recognize Alice and greet her. Her new class also had monthly field trips into the community. It was at this school that Alice's personality really started to shine. She was happy most of the time and it showed in her interaction and reaction to the experiences at her school and extra-curricular activities.

With the support of her new class, Alice was working on her augmented communication device and she began testing on a self-propelled wheelchair. There was also a specialized tricycle that Carol used around the neighborhood. Alice used a supportive seat. Her feet were secured by Velcro to the pedals and, with Carol's assistance, she would bicycle around the neighborhood. She could pedal herself a little bit and when she got tired Carol would push the bike which would move the pedal for Alice passively. She loved riding on the bike. Disco came along which was always interesting because Disco liked to take her time walking and had to sniff everything. Carol would "yell" at Disco to get moving and Alice would laugh. In the afternoons after school or on weekends, using her communication device, Alice chose what activity she wanted to do after her snack and before dinner. Choices included reading books, listening to music (Carol would lay Alice on the ground stretched out while she was listening), swinging in her backyard swing, playing games, jumping on the trampoline or bike riding. There was a large specialty swing which was hanging on the swing set that Alice enjoyed using. She also loved the trampoline. Carol would stand behind her supporting her. Then they would jump up and down together. She loved it but it was tiring for Carol. Then Carol would lay her down and either jump around her so she bounced around a bit or, if G3 and his friends were there, they would often "help" by jumping carefully around her. Then she would sit on the edge with Carol on the ground standing behind her while the boys jumped on the trampoline vigorously. Alice enjoyed watching them and she could get a little bounce while sitting too.

Carol also, for many years, took Alice to the town pools in the summer. There was a wading pool. Carol would hold her and help her in the water, which, in a wading pool, is not too easy on one's back. Carol met several Moms at the wading pool who were not put off by the wheelchair and who became friends. One young Mom was a single mother dealing with an autistic son. Another family had a daughter the same age as Alice and a son who became one of G3's best friends. That relationship was started over Thomas the Tank engine trains. G3 brought the trains to the wading pool and chugged his trains on the side of the pool attracting the attention of another young preschooler who loved trains as well. The Mom was a special education teacher. G3 and the other young boy turned out to be in the same preschool class and the families of each became fast friends.

Alice was older and heavier when the family moved to the new house and Carol took Alice to the town park pool. The town pool handicapped entrance was on the far side of the pool, so they had to check in and then push Alice on the outside of the building down a sidewalk to meet a lifeguard by the entrance. The lifeguard would unlock the door; they would enter and then have to walk back from the deep end to the shallow end where the ramp into the pool was. By then, just about everyone in and out of the pool would be looking for them. If one has a child with a disability, one better not be self-conscious or have confidence issues. Carol would then have to place the wheelchair at the top of the ramp and carry Alice into the pool or out of the pool when they were finished. The public pools always had a lot of activity which attracted Alice's attention. Usually there would be a young girl or another parent who was interested in Alice and would talk with her. Over the next few summers, Alice got to be very heavy and virtually impossible to carry in and out of the pool. Finally, the Andersons decided to put a pool in their backyard with a lift. The pool was great, a lot easier, but Carol did miss all the activity at the public pools. When G3's friends were swimming in the pool, Alice was always thrilled. The lift made getting her in and out of the pool easier and made a swim a lot less stressful for Carol without having to load all of the equipment and strap Alice into and out of the van as well.

In the wintertime, Alice kept swimming by going to a large indoor town pool where Carol worked. Over time, Carol had moved from taking aerobic classes to teaching them. Becoming an aerobics instructor and later a personal trainer was a great part time job for her because she was able to make a little extra money doing a job which she could work around her schedule with the kids. The pool had a lift and gave Alice some exercise in the winter on days off from school. With traveling, clothing changes took a lot of time and effort, but Alice enjoyed it and movement was good for her. G3 would often bring a friend with him which made it fun for him, too.

Nighttime usually involved Daddy-time for Alice. Greg would often get her ready for bed although Carol often assisted. Greg and Alice got into the habit of listening to Doctor Laura on the radio while Greg was bathing and getting Alice ready for the night. It was fun to listen to Alice laugh sometimes at Dr. Laura's voice or comments. Someone always read Alice a book or two before bed and then put her into her specialty bed. Daddy had his routine to say good night while Carol would sing her a song and rub her back or arm before lights out.

Chapter 6

Disco

Dr. Anderson retired to Florida in July 1997. He and Millie had realized a bit of money from the sale of the house up north, in the high rent district, and so they were able to build a lovely home on the golf course in a town near Tampa, Florida. They already had numerous social friends in the area and so had no trouble establishing themselves in the new place. The main problem seemed to be that now they were farther away from the children and grandchildren than they had been.

Alice was six years old. The Anderson's lanai featured a large pool, warm year round. Alice's shouts of glee when she was in the pool were music to their ears.

Shortly after they moved, their youngest son, Andy and his wife, Pat, drove the Anderson's second car to Florida. As yet, these two did not have children. But they did have a dog—in fact Andy and Pat had both grown up with dogs so it seemed natural to them that Andy's parents should have one, too.

A look through the want ads produced information about a basset hound breeder just then selling puppies, recently weaned. Robert and Millie Anderson knew that one does not go to see adorable puppies without buying one! But they went anyway, with the kids and were introduced to a beautiful female puppy.

Now, their eldest son and his family had a basset named Duchess. The elder Andersons had already decided on a "royal" name for a new dog, but did not want to out-rank Duchess. And so they decided that Countess would be appropriate. As the sale was concluded, the breeder gave them a bit off of the puppy price. Countess immediately became "disCountess". Her street name then became "Disco".

Luckily the new house had tile walkways between carpeted areas leading to both sides of the house. Disco's response when someone would come to the door was to rush there, nails clicking on the tiles, turn over on her back and pee up. The Anderson's friends soon became adjusted to this procedure and so Disco spent very little time in her pen except at night or when the house was empty.

Having had dogs all their lives, one would think that the Andersons would understand what a responsibility a dog, especially a new, young one, would be. The children went home and their folks were left to deal with Disco. She really was a lovely animal and the Andersons were at pains to educate themselves about basset hounds.

After a little while, however, Disco began to impact her owners' freedom in retirement. Frequent interruptions of social events happened because Disco needed attending to, with a little early rising and some noise soon gave them to realize that perhaps they had made a mistake acquiring a dog. What to do about that was the next problem.

A telephone call to daughter Jayne and her husband Jacob in North Carolina to see if they wanted a dog was made. These two said yes, they would love to have Disco, but that Alice's father and mother had recently told them that they were thinking about acquiring a dog for Alice and her brother.

So the next call was to Greg and Carol. Yes, they said, they would love to have Disco. (By this time all the Anderson children and grandchildren had met Disco.)

So the arrangements were made to ship Disco to them. Robert then became the only person in their social circle who had actually been to the Air Transport section of Tampa International Airport. By the time the shipping requirements and air fare were met, it cost $400.00 to fly Disco to her new home. As Robert was saying goodbye to Disco, he noticed that he was surrounded by large crates. He asked what they were. They were coffins. He should have known.

As he left the loading area he noticed that two of the airline workers were already playing with Disco as best they could through the wire of her pen.

Disco survived the trip (some 20% of animals shipped by air do not survive the journey) and the Andersons settled down to once again enjoy their serenity. To be honest, they suspected that their friends were happy not to have to deal with Disco any more, either.

Disco proved to be a wonderful animal for Alice and her brother. They would lie on the floor with their heads on Disco's belly to watch television. Alice would squeal when Disco licked her. Her grown-up owners kept the dog scrupulously clean. She had her own living area in the large laundry room as well as a good-sized pen outdoors with direct access from the garage. Alice's father, with help from her brother, built a large doghouse for Disco. It only took the dog two years to finally use the house. Until then she would stay out of the rain under the eaves of the Anderson's house and curl up there when the weather was inclement or even snowing. Whenever the elder Andersons would arrive for a visit, Disco immediately remembered them. Later when she was very old she probably remembered them by their scents.

When Alice was about three years old and had outgrown her crib, her parents purchased a very special bed for her. Quite expensive. It had nylon mesh sides; the mesh strands were flat and slightly curved. Their edges were not sharp or very hard. Shortly after Alice began using the bed, during one night, Disco was heard barking which she almost never did. Upon investigation, Greg found that Alice had gotten into a position, by chance, which was up against the nylon mesh. Unable to control her involuntary movements, she suffered damage to her skin where it had been rubbing against the mesh. No one will ever know why Disco was alerted to this problem, but, had she not sounded the warning, Alice might have sustained far more damage than she did. She healed quickly and Disco was now and forever a heroine. (Much more about this particular model of her bed is revealed later in Alice's story.)

Disco got to be a very large dog eventually. She was rarely sick. Finally, however, she did lose her eyesight and then her hearing. Nevertheless she still knew when someone was getting ice cubes, which she loved, out of the refrigerator and was always able to find the patch of sunlight that shone in through the door to the patio. And she would always roll over to have her tummy rubbed, even though it took her longer and longer to do so.

Finally, rather than have her be in pain from several other ailments, Disco had to be "put down". Millie Anderson cried when she heard the news, and the rest of the family was sad, too. Disco was twelve years old by then and had contributed much to their family. Even though Alice's father always referred to Disco as "the goddamned dog", we all knew he loved her, too, and appreciated the comfort the dog had provided for Alice and the family.

Disco was the perfect dog for the family. She was very calm, slept all day and was very "low need". So much of the Anderson's time was spent taking care of Alice, that the family needed a dog like Disco who required little attention. When Disco got excited and did laps around the house, Alice would laugh so hard she would almost have trouble breathing.

Chapter 7

Alice's House

A short while after Alice's brother Greg (G3) was born, as a result of the malpractice lawsuit in which part of the settlement money was to be used for a new house, the Andersons were able to build a place to live suited to Alice's needs as well as equipment for Alice to use. They were able to build in such a way that it did not appear to be a "handicapped" house at all. There are no significant door sills or transitions between rooms. The halls are wider than normal to accommodate a wheelchair. There is tile and wood and low-nap carpeting on the floors where one might expect. Since Alice's parents had the large van for ease of transporting their daughter, they had the garage doors made taller than normal. There are steps, but all are associated with ramps which are done in concrete. Exiting onto the patio, one can go down several stairs to a larger lower level or walk around a small garden featuring a lovely red maple tree and down a slightly inclined ramp to the lower level.

Alice's en suite bathroom was outfitted with an enormous shower capable of accommodating her wheel-chair. A roll-under sink with a mirror which is easily adjusted to different heights is present. The bathroom itself is large also, to make room for easy accessibility. The roll-in shower made bathing her so much easier. An almost level transfer from her wheelchair to the changing table plus an easy transfer to a high rolling shower chair made the nighttime routine convenient.

All of the light switches in the house are at a slightly lower level than normal, roller switches, but, like the other adjustments this is not immediately apparent.

Eventually a lovely heated, securely fenced, in-ground pool appeared in the back yard.

Alice loved being in the water and her father never seemed to tire of playing with her on her "noodles". She didn't mind in the least feeling cold when she came out of the water—she just wanted to "swim" some more. In the winter, at the elder Anderson's house in Florida, she got some extra time in the water. Alice got to use a new pool lift at her house for the summer it was installed. The lift at her house eased her transition into the water. Gregory and Carol never regretted this pool work, because it had been for Alice.

The new house made a lot of things easier and convenient and the Andersons did a lot of research to make it work for them. Alice actually got to the point of being able to reach for a switch and switching it on or off occasionally, with encouragement. Some other equipment such as the shower chair, changing table and pool lift were available for Alice. When Alice was younger, her parents tried to get insurance to pay for a shower chair for her. The insurance company denied the request saying it was not medically necessary, a decision Carol would never understand. How could it not be medically necessary to keep one's child clean? Not to mention that without a bathing chair, the caregivers were much more likely to suffer an injury, probably to the back. Issues from not being clean or an injured back would have been much more expensive for the insurance company than just getting the simple adaptive chair. In addition, a huge help after the settlement was the ability to purchase vans with wheelchair lifts.

When the elder Andersons moved into their new house in Delaware, they installed a fountain in the form of a castle complete with a moat. It was placed in a square garden just outside the front door. A sign there indicates that this is "Allie's Castle". People coming and going always want to have this memorial explained to them. It also carries on Alice's love

Part II

"Blessed are they who mourn, for they shall be comforted."

Matthew 5:4

Preliminary Statement

A memorandum prepared by the Anderson's Lawyers prior to legal proceedings.

"The whole is greater than the sum of its parts." The tight-knit (Anderson) family knows the truth of this statement and embodies it. Each activity in which one member of the family is involved becomes a gathering point for the rest of the family. Whether Alice's horseback riding, ice skating, or dancing, or Greg III's baseball, soccer or band, each activity is an opportunity to spend time together as a family and to support each other. The (Anderson) family is better together than apart. That is why whoever meets the Andersons or even just one member of the family instantly knows how strong, supportive and loving a family they are.

This memorandum offers some insight into the lives of the (Anderson) family and illustrates their collective efforts to create this close-knit family that amazes and inspires those they meet.

Greg and Carol met while both were attending University.

After dating through college, they knew their lives were better with each other than without. They married on August 1, 1987 with a dream of starting a family together.

In 1991, their dream came true. They found out that Carol was pregnant, and, on May 13, 1991, Carol gave birth to their first child, Alice. Alice was a wonderful gift of love. She was born with cerebral palsy, but Alice's disability never slowed her down. Nor did it slow down Greg and Carol. Having a child with C.P. made them realize how fragile life can be, and how lucky they were to have a child at all. As a result, they made sure that Alice received the best medical treatment possible. (This is attested to by a letter from Alice's pediatrician describing Greg and Carol's efforts to provide the best care for Alice.)

Greg and Carol's love for Alice was about more than just making her comfortable and healthy. They wanted Alice to love life and feel loved. They helped Alice to be involved in as many activities as possible. Beginning at a very young age, Alice was involved in the Skating Association for the Blind and Handicapped. Alice was also involved in horseback riding, challenger softball, and Moving Miracles, a dance class for children with disabilities. Greg and Carol were extremely active in encouraging these pursuits for Alice. Carol volunteered with ice skating and became a Board member with Moving Miracles. Greg coached Alice's softball team.

In 1993, the (Anderson) family grew again. Carol, Greg and Alice welcomed Gregory III into their home. Alice and G3 grew very close and shared a special bond. Theirs was a unique relationship; Alice was both a big sister and a kid sister to G3. He watched over Alice like a younger sister, but admired her for the gentle older sibling she was.

As both Alice and G3 grew, Greg and Carol's involvement in their children's growth and development increased as well. G3 became involved in baseball, soccer, Boy Scouts, and playing the trombone. Alice's activities increased as she learned to ski, swim and bowl. Each activity in which Alice or G3 became involved became a family activity. Either Carol or Greg (or both) would try to take a leadership role in the activity (coaching, advising, or volunteering), and the other members of the family became vocal cheerleaders. For example, when G3 became involved in Boy Scouts, Greg became a leader on the parents' committee. Alice served as the Grand Marshall to the Boy Scouts' Pinewood Derby Race while Carol cheered on as a proud parent of her two children.

Greg and Carol also broadened their children's horizons through travel. The family traveled throughout the country together. Alice loved roller coasters, so the Andersons traveled to Hershey, Pennsylvania, Cedar

Point, Ohio, and Florida to various amusement parks. They also traveled to New York, Florida, Delaware and other destinations to visit their large extended family.

The closeness of the family inspired family and friends who had the pleasure of witnessing their special bond. In sympathy cards and letters sent to the Andersons after the tragic passing of Alice, people commented on how close they are and how their love for each other was evident in their lives.

The (Andersons) demonstrated to everyone they met that their closeness as a family enabled them to conquer any obstacle life threw at them and enjoy every precious moment together.

Chapter 1

Alice Dies

Robert and Millie Anderson were a little sad driving home from church on May 2, 2004, a warm Sunday morning in Florida. It was the last time they would attend Mass at St. Clement's Church until they were, perhaps, visiting in the area. They and many others had contributed to the construction of this large, modern, beautiful, Spanish-style structure. They had many friends among the parishioners, staff and religious there and had been inspired by the people they met and the activities they participated in.

The following day, the movers would be arriving to pack up for the trip to a new house up north near their youngest son, Andy, and his family. Robert would have his last appointment with his podiatrist and good friend and then they would be off to yet another new life.

The telephone was flashing when they arrived home with a message from Greg to call him. Millie did so immediately while Robert was standing nearby. It was then that Greg delivered the news that Alice was dead. Millie's reaction indicated to Robert that the news was awful, and without talking to Greg he knew that one of Greg's two children had died. Millie was weeping and Robert screamed out, "Which one?" To say that Robert lost it then would be to drastically understate his reaction. All he could think of was that a moment before he had had six beautiful grandchildren and now he had only five. Millie, having an excess of patience and being always better at these kinds of things, listened as Greg said he would call back and then hung up. The Andersons tried to comfort one another, but Robert's reaction was so over the top that it was difficult to do. They held onto one another and cried inconsolably.

Almost immediately, the telephone began to ring—the other children and then friends from all over were calling. Things were beginning to be under a little better control, while Millie gracefully accepted their concern, saying that she had no details whatsoever, and they would soon be in touch.

By the time Millie had called to tell their nearest friends the news, Robert had begun to recover a bit as his shock dissipated. And then the doorbell began to ring. Everyone in their crowd had come to know Alice during her frequent visits to her grandparents. They came to express their grief and to be sure that the Andersons were holding up. Robert has no recollection of eating that day. To their dismay, there were some who did not seem able to understand the problems they faced just then; their bereavement, the moving plans, and certain health issues.

Robert knew that it wasn't necessary for him to cancel his doctor appointment since the doctor would hear what had happened almost immediately. It was Sunday and so there remained the appointment with the moving people the next day to deal with, since the company could not be reached.

At midnight, Millie managed to arrange for them to fly out at noon the next day. A long-time dear friend and neighbor drove them to the airport.

The moving people were ultra-cooperative in rescheduling the move on such short notice.

In The City, Millie and Robert met their oldest son, Robert, Jr., at the airport just after he had arrived from Houston, Texas. Alice's other grandfather, Henry MacDowell, arrived to pick up all three and take them to the Anderson's house in Maneta. It was a very unhappy ride for all.

It was also a quiet ride to Greg and Carol's house—the Anderson's were glad to have their son along. They knew he would be support for his brother Greg and for them as well.

Henry then delivered the next shock—the police were investigating Alice's death.

Arriving at the Anderson's house in the early evening of May 3, Alice's two grandfathers, Grammy and Uncle, Robert, Jr., were met with a crowd of people, mostly coming and going, often laden with food; a good thing since there were so many people around. Of course, greeting Greg and Carol and G3 was heart-breaking for all. The death of anyone is usually a sad occasion, but the tragedy of a child lost is almost unbearable.

Following are events of the early days in May 2004:

Saturday, May 1, 2004 had been a busy day for Alice and her parents. This was not unusual, given the time it took to prepare Alice for her many daily activities. This always included Alice's stretching exercises. Greg gave Alice her medications. Since Carol was at the YMCA completing a Continuing Education Unit, Alice's father drove her to her horseback riding and dance programs. She was wearing a short sleeve shirt this day since it was warm and Alice became more limp when she was too warm. She wore a vest and helmet when she rode. Greg needed assistance with the two-person lift used to set Alice upon her horse. The session lasted 30 minutes.

Then it was off to the dance program at Moving Miracles where G3 helped his father ready Alice for the program. Her activity this day was difficult for Alice, but she persevered and completed it. Then, Greg dropped G3 off at a friend's birthday party and returned home to clean Alice up and have lunch. After lunch, Carol and Alice went for a bike ride, the bike specially fitted for Alice, and they returned home in the afternoon in time to go to church at 5:00 pm.

Three Andersons went out to dinner this evening, during which they received from the birthday boy's mother a call that her son had broken his collarbone and she was taking all the boys to the hospital to have her son checked. The Andersons arrived at the hospital shortly thereafter—the birthday boy's parents knew Alice and commented on how she had grown and how mature she looked now and how nice her haircut was.

After getting home, Carol and Greg got Alice ready for bed; they gave her an acetaphenamin suppository because she had a slight fever, 100.4 degrees. Then Greg put Alice in bed, rolling her to the right side facing the wall. He adjusted her legs and arms to a comfortable position with a pillow under her head, arms to the right and legs slightly separated to avoid sores. He then said "Goodnight" to Alice by "snuggling" with her so he could receive her open-mouthed kiss. Carol did the same thing—Greg could hear the kisses over the intercom. After that it was time for G3 to go to bed. Carol could hear this procedure over the intercom so she went to G3's room to say, "Goodnight". Later, Greg and Carol watched TV for a short while and then went to bed themselves. Carol checked on G3, but not Alice since doing so would have startled her awake. The monitor was on in Alice's room.

Carol and Greg slept through the night, neither having had to get up to care for Alice, although Carol thought she might have heard Alice make a noise during the night, but she was not sure and it did not continue.

Carol and Greg then had coffee in the family room and, at 9:00 am on May 2, Greg went to check on Alice. The late hour was not unusual for them on a weekend morning. When he opened Alice's door, he did not notice the "startle" that always occurred with Alice when her door was opened. He knew immediately that something was wrong. He went to the side of her bed calling, "Good morning, Allie" and looking for movement of the blanket and comforter that covered her. He expected movement as he lowered the usually noisy side rail and unzipped the safety net. He called her name, throwing the blankets off of her. He then reached across the bed to get her. She was lying with her head to the right facing toward the wall. The pillow was touching the top of her head. Her torso was twisted with her left shoulder facing Greg, her left arm at her side and her left-hand on her buttock. He put his hands underneath her; her legs were slightly bent with her knees toward the wall. Greg could see the back of her head by her left ear.

The head of the bed was elevated and her head was not on the pillow. Greg then pulled Alice's entire body toward him. She was blue. Her left hand was blue and she was not breathing while Greg checked for a pulse. As he pulled her to the side of the bed where he stood, he screamed for Carol and screamed Alice's name. Upon entering the room, Carol shouted to G3 to call

911. Greg continued to check Alice for breathing and a pulse and clearing mucus from her nostrils by squeezing her nose from bridge to tip.

Carol retrieved the phone, gave it to Greg and began CPR. While listening to 911 instructions on CPR, Greg told G3 to remain by the front door to direct the EMTs. Greg and Carol were alternating CPR by now, and, when the EMT arrived, they expected that he would take over. The EMT instructed Greg to place Alice on the floor and continue with CPR chest compression. Another EMT then took over as the first EMT unsuccessfully tried to place a breathing tube in Alice's airway. He finally was successful in doing this. A mask was placed which fit over Alice's entire head because of the small size of her head. Then Greg was asked to leave the room so as to make space for all the EMTs.

Arriving in the foyer, Greg encountered the county sheriff and a state trooper at the entrance. Shortly, the EMTs wheeled Alice out on a gurney, face up, covered neck to toe, no CPR being done, no oxygen being administered, and placed her in the EMTs' vehicle. Carol was not allowed to ride to the hospital with Alice. The state police took Carol to the hospital while Greg got his things, locked up the house and took G3 to a friend's house. During the ride Carol asked why the ambulance was not flashing lights. At the house, a man, not in uniform, was completing a report asking only for Greg's name, phone number and address. No other details for the report were asked for nor stated by Greg.

At the hospital he was directed to the family waiting room where Carol had been taken. They held each other and cried. After a few minutes, a doctor and a nurse came in and explained that Alice had died. The doctor noted that Alice had been dead for some time. Then, her parents were allowed to spend time with Allie. In the room where Alice lay, Greg noticed the tube that had been inserted, blood on her teeth and gums, a dark bruise on her nose and a similar bruise on her right jawbone. This was the first time Greg had seen these markings.

The pastoral minister came to the room. They described Alice's beautiful personality to him and prayed. Greg cried to the point of having a nose bleed. The pair left the room with the minster. Alice had been wearing her "star" pajamas, Carol remembered. The Andersons left the hospital to pick up G3 and returned home.

Chapter 2

Police Investigations

As the day moved on, many people had arrived at the Anderson's house, and more continued to arrive during that day and the next, including grandparents, Anderson siblings, Carol's sister, Roselyn, and Greg and Carol's friends. Robert, Jr. eventually took Millie and Robert to their motel, and they were able to get a little rest, having slept poorly the night after Alice died and not at all on their trip to Maneta. In the morning, Tuesday, May 4, they returned to their children's house, little suspecting what was about to happen.

In the afternoon of May 4, two police officers who were familiar with Greg and Carol, having interviewed them earlier in the day at the house, indicated that Alice's parents should accompany them to the police barracks. They told the Andersons that they did not need to be represented by a lawyer at that time. They were told that the medical examiner had an idea about what had happened, an idea that later stunned Robert, a practicing physician. However, the police would not divulge this "idea".

At the barracks, a male and a female police officer interviewed Carol. The female officer left the room first followed later by the male officer. Carol was left by herself and she could hear Greg crying at that time in the room next door. In the brief time she was alone, Carol realized what was happening. She left the room and went to find her father, Henry, who had driven the Andersons to the police station and who had been in the waiting room the whole time. He was worried listening to what the police were saying outside the interviewing rooms. Her father reinforced Carol's realization that the Andersons were about to be accused of killing Alice. Carol then went back to the room Greg was in and interrupted. She told Greg that they were being accused of murdering Alice and that there had been enough questioning of them both and that they were leaving. Carol felt that she had to protect her husband and her son quickly, and that they needed an attorney.

The police had asked probing questions such as, did one or the other of the parents smother Alice with a pillow case, had Alice put up a struggle? Greg was required to take off his shirt to show that he did not have any defensive wounds on him. Greg later said that he was left sitting there trying to get through this incredible grief while the police were thinking that he murdered his daughter.

The Andersons, too, wanted to know how Alice had died. Long before any investigation was complete, the county medical examiner had decided that Alice died of asphyxia and that she would eventually check homicide on the death certificate. This fit nicely with the examiner's theory, which she had espoused publicly; that a death occurring at home, especially of a handicapped person, was murder! This was the "idea", the police had referred to. To Dr. Anderson, this was so utterly far-fetched as to be ludicrous.

The state police supervisor later said that, based on the facts that they had received, they were obligated to thoroughly investigate the circumstances of her death.

Meanwhile, while Greg and Carol were at the police station, at home Grandmother Helga MacDowell, "Omi" to the grandchildren, became increasingly upset about the length of time the Andersons were being kept. And rightly so.

As Carol's father, Henry MacDowell, was driving them home, the Andersons called their family lawyer who gave them a referral to the attorneys that they eventually worked with. By the time they called, the police had already gone into the house without a search warrant.

When Greg and Carol finally arrived back home, they found a black van in their driveway, presumably from the state police to carry away evidence, and, of all things, a K-9 unit parked across the street. Most alarming of all was the white Central Police Services vehicle parked across the street. Also, one can only imagine the neighbors' reaction. Henry, while waiting for the Andersons at the police barracks, had overheard conversations which included talk of calling Child Protective Services (CPS) because of the remaining child, George III, in the house.

Shortly, the state police arrived and quickly interviewed Greg and Carol. In the house, they followed everyone around, even following Robert to the bathroom. The lawyer, "Vince", was quickly on site. He forced the issue of the need for a search warrant on the police. But, they would not leave the house. Then, before the search warrant arrived, Vince, who was to do such excellent work for the family in the future, thought it best to interview the Andersons in his car because of all the people and all the confusion in the house.

A search warrant finally arrived, whereupon the police emptied out Alice's room, bed and all, and even included the laundry room (for which they did not have a warrant). One law enforcement official was heard to say, "The police believe that someone in this house killed Alice."

After much discussion with the attorney, and because of the Anderson's fears that their son would be traumatized if his parents were arrested in front of him, and with all of the police in the house, as well as fears that CPS would attempt to remove him, the Andersons decided to have Carol's parents take him somewhere safe. (Thinking back on this still causes a visceral reaction in Carol many years later.)

It was at this point, as Robert was standing outside, that Henry and Helga appeared with G3 and headed to their car. He asked where they were going and, when Henry said that they were going to get some supper, Robert offered to go along. Whereupon, Henry quietly replied that they were going out to supper in East Vale. This is where they lived, about 250 miles from Maneta. Then they drove off, Robert quietly cheering them on. They were followed by a state police car. The police tailed them for about 100 miles before giving up following them. The police did not try to stop them.

By this time, both of the Andersons were frightened to go anywhere; leaving the other at home alone raising the possibility that the police might come to arrest that person.

Both were unable to be alone together in the house as well, for a similar reason. Every time they left the house, they were petrified that upon returning home the police would be at the door or in the driveway with arrest warrants. Carol was so worried that G3 was going to lose not only his sister but both parents as well that she actually lost 15 pounds in eight days. (Carol has no extra pounds on her frame to actually lose, but, at this time, she really did lose weight.) This despite all the food that people were bringing in!

Adding to the emotional trauma of all this was that visiting hours and Alice's funeral were already scheduled when the Andersons were told by the funeral director that Alice's body would not be released yet. Many of their friends showed up at the funeral home only to find a sign on the door saying that the schedule was cancelled and no new date was available. When Alice's body was finally released, the funeral director had to take Alice to an out of town neighboring medical center for a third autopsy, arranged by the Anderson's attorney to establish the cause of death. So, the funeral was delayed for over a week. By that time the Andersons thought they could only endure one day of visiting hours. For that, the line of friends and relatives extended out of the door of the funeral home. Carol would later find that even more people were not able to be present, many having come to visiting hours which subsequently were cancelled.

The Anderson's daughter, Aunt Joyce, arrived on Thursday, May 6; Uncle Robert, Jr. left on Friday. Greg indicated to his brother that he did not need to return for Alice's funeral because, at the time that Robert, Jr. left, no one had any idea when the service would take place.

Andrew Anderson, wife Patricia and their daughter Caroline also arrived later from Delaware for the funeral, while Caroline's brother was being cared for by his "other" grandparents. He was too young to attend the funeral.

A complaint to the sheriff's department was later filed by Carol and Greg with regard to events noted above, is quoted here:

"The purpose of this letter is to file a complaint with your department. Our daughter, Alice, died on the morning of May 2, 2004 at our residence in the town of Maneta. The actions, or lack thereof on the part of the sheriff's department on that day and the days immediately following her death are the substance of this complaint.

On the morning of May 2, our daughter was found unresponsive in her Vail safety bed. A 911 phone call was made at approximately 9 am. Paramedics, a county sheriff's officer and a State Police officer responded to our call for help. After local emergency medical personnel attempted to resuscitate Alice, she was transported to the local suburban hospital where she was pronounced dead. Before Alice was taken to the hospital, neither the sheriff's officer nor the state trooper made any attempt to take jurisdiction, secure the scene or investigate so that the cause and manner of death could be determined. Neither police agency took a detailed statement at our home or the hospital. We were informed by the hospital's attending clergy that the medical examiner would do an autopsy on the following day.

On the afternoon of the following day, we were told by Alice's funeral director that the medical examiner would not release our daughter until an autopsy was completed the following day. After several calls to the sheriff's office and the state police, we were told that the autopsy had been delayed due to jurisdictional indecision between the sheriff's department and the state police. Thirty six hours after Alice's death, it became apparent that the state police had gained jurisdiction.

With this letter, we allege that the initial failure of the responding agencies to quickly determine jurisdiction and fully and properly investigate the matter immediately following the death of our daughter caused our family and ourselves an immeasurable amount of emotional distress and legal fees to sort out the resulting chaos.

We further allege that the failure of the sheriff's department to determine jurisdiction quickly, complete a thorough investigation and provide the medical examiner with accurate, definitive and complete information, resulted in an incorrect determination of the manner of death. Therefore, we request that this matter be investigated and that appropriate disciplinary action be taken against the members of the sheriff's department who were involved. This would include interviews of the first responders as well as consideration of the possibility of consultation with a polygraph expert."

Later, the Andersons contemplated suing both agencies.

A similar complaint was filed with the state police. This complaint contained more details, some described here:

While at the Anderson's house, neither the sheriff nor the state police officer made any inquiries of the Andersons, nor did they secure the scene of Alice's death. While at the hospital, the Andersons were asked a few basic questions such as their names, address and the fact that Alice had cerebral palsy. The officer took no detailed statement from them.

After the state police officially took jurisdiction, two officers, both Investigators, arrived at the Anderson's residence. The female investigator took a detailed, several pages long statement from Carol. The male officer wrote out a statement of one paragraph from Greg after speaking with him for almost an hour. This officer also took photos of the bed. This investigation was occurring beyond 36 hours after the death of the Anderson's daughter and the material information from the scene of her death had changed, including information that it was imperative to have in determining the proper cause of Alice's death.

After the Andersons were informed by the funeral home director that the medical examiner was holding their daughter, two more investigators arrived asking Greg and Carol to come to the state police station on Main Street in town. The police were aware that the Andersons had an attorney representing them since the attorney had made several phone calls to the sheriff and the state police on their behalf to iron out the jurisdictional issues of the previous day. The Andersons asked at this time if their attorney should be present and were advised by the officers that they would not need an attorney.

At the police station as noted above, both Andersons were questioned at length without their attorney present. At this time they were accused of killing their daughter. Carol and Greg were questioned separately. Carol told the questioning officers that her daughter was found in a position in the bed which she could not get out of. Greg, also questioned by two investigators, repeatedly advised the questioners that Alice's bed was involved. The tone of the questioning was accusative rather than information-seeking. The officers never investigated further the important information regarding the bed that had been given to them, nor did they pass the information along to the medical examiner. They also refused to answer questions as to the results of the autopsy which would have enabled them to present information about the Vail bed in which Alice slept.

In mid-afternoon, immediately after returning to their home after the questioning, the state police arrived en masse. Carol asked if they had a search warrant to enter the house. The officers stated that they were in the process of obtaining one. Carol then refused to allow them access to the residence, whereupon she was told to "quiet down and let them (the police) do their jobs". Then, about six officers entered by way of the front door. The Andersons, not wanting to make a bad situation worse and feeling powerless to stop them, let the police in. The state police then seized control of the house, with several officers in the front hall guarding the front door, officers guarding the door from the laundry room to the garage, officers in the bedroom hallway and in Alice's room and the driveway. The police presence included a canine unit with a dog maliciously barking non-stop except when its officer let the dog run to relieve itself on the neighbor's lawn. About an hour after all of this, the Anderson's attorney arrived.

The police refused to leave the premises at the request of the Anderson's attorney.

The search warrant was finally obtained 4½ hours later which allowed for the search of Alice's bedroom only, though there were police in most of the rooms of the house. Finally, the police dismantled Alice's bed. However, they never reconstructed it as part of the investigation, further destroying important evidence because it was, in fact, the specialty Vail bed that was the cause of her death. An investigation of the scene immediately upon Alice's death would have shown that she had been found in her bed in an unusual position that was the result of entrapment in the bed. A simple internet search by the investigating officers would have revealed similar problems with the bed, eliminating over two years of pain and suffering on the part of the family.

Many family members were in the house at this time, including both sets of Alice's grandparents, two of Greg's siblings and ten year old G3, who by now, like everyone else had undergone a great deal of emotional trauma.

In this complaint, the Andersons also alleged that the initial failure of the responding agencies to determine jurisdiction quickly and to investigate immediately, fully and properly the circumstances of Alice's death, caused their family and themselves an immeasurable amount of emotional distress and over $80,000 in legal fees to straighten out the resulting problems. Also, because the medical examiner did not have the correct information when she conducted her autopsy, she reached an incorrect determination of the manner of death. This resulted, again, in necessary legal action and over two years of emotional upheaval.

The Andersons also further alleged that their civil rights were violated when they were questioned without an attorney present. The civil rights of all the people present in their house were also violated (under Article 6 of the Bill of Rights) because their freedom of movement was restricted and all had been detained. As a result of the complaint filed, the state police sent an officer to investigate. He asked questions. A transcript of the conversation was provided upon the Anderson's request. This forms the basis of the questions and answers described below. While the state police found no wrongful actions on the Anderson's part, Greg and Carol were at least able to their express their feelings to a representative. The sheriff's department never contacted them.

Chapter 3

Autopsies

Alice's remains underwent three autopsies. Authorization was given to disclose to the Andersons any examination or autopsy records or reports pertaining to Alice.

The first autopsy was done by the county medical examiner, Dr. Wyman, in consultation with her colleague in New York City. At the outset, it should be noted that Dr. Wyman had previously publicly stated that any death of a disabled person at home was due to non-accidental cause. Her colleague had published a paper in NYC based on a study of 26 patients in a city of 8 million people, entitled "The Importance of Cerebral Palsy in the Manner of Death", wherein she states, "proper reporting and investigation of these deaths is required for accurate certification of the cause and manner of death . . . ."

The medical examiner found no signs of disease in Alice, except for the external marks on her body after resuscitation efforts, and petechiae associated with her eyes.

Dr. Wyman concluded that "the cause of death of this 12 year old Caucasian female child is Asphyxia due to Compression of the Neck. Contributing factors are a history of cerebral palsy related to perinatal asphyxia. Following a complete autopsy including a review of birth reports, medical reports, state police reports and photographs, the manner of death is Homicide".

The medical examiner was aware of Alice's physical activities, and that she had a Baclofen pump implanted (resulting in minimal contractures of her extremities). She also knew of Alice's history of seizures and her disability in rolling over. The police also noted that "the parents had monitors all over the house just because they were afraid she could get into trouble".

The pediatrician carefully explained to the medical examiner how severe Alice's cerebral palsy was. He said that, through the efforts of her parents, she was much better off than many children with her degree of CP.

The pediatrician also felt that Dr. Wyman was being very vague in describing her own investigation. He did not know whether this was because the investigation was incomplete at this point or if she was deliberately vague to try to draw the pediatrician out.

Dr. Wyman sent her findings relating to Alice's autopsy to Dr. Sumpter in New York City.

She agreed with Dr. Wyman stating, "I have concluded that the cause of death is "Compression of the Neck" and the manner of death is "Homicide". Please let me know if I can be of further assistance."

The second autopsy was done at the request of the state police. The district attorney asked the state police to request an autopsy outside of Dr. Wyman's office because the district attorney was not confident in the original autopsy. In this case, the examining pathologist gave the following opinion:

"I have performed a 'second autopsy' on the remains of Alice Anderson at the county medical examiner's office at the request of the state police. I have also reviewed the investigative reports, certain documents of the past medical examination history, and interviews obtained by the police from relevant parties along with the original autopsy report of Dr. Wyman, her sixty microscopic slides on the case and numerous on scene and autopsy photographs. It is my opinion that the cause of death is not definitively revealed by the autopsy and related materials. Although certain small hemorrhages in the tissues of the neck may suggest an asphyxial homicide, the history of resuscitation by at least three successive lay and professional parties on a deceased individual with rigor and livor and the observation of petechiae most numerous below the neck suggest to me that these extravasations of blood may be artifactual and/or misleading. The death may well be due to seizure and there is a history of seizure disorder as part of her cerebral palsy. The copious edema in her airway (Photo #4 in my Group III-dated 5/4) and the lack of petechiae there suggest seizure activity. Airway obstruction by mucus is another possibility. The activities of the day included one care-giver being alarmed at her breathing sounds. Significant mucus was described during the "resuscitation" efforts. I am therefore unable to agree that this case is a homicide and consider the manner to also be 'undetermined'".

The third autopsy was done at the behest of Alice's parents by a pathologist in a university medical school setting in a nearby city. ("We would like to retain you and your office to conduct a post-mortem examination of Alice.") The work product included authorization for the out-of county medical examiner to do a post-mortem examination and to share and discuss the results of the examination with the Anderson's attorney.

Terms of the agreement for examination above also were included.

The Anderson's attorneys are to be notified if: the exhibition or surrender of any documents or records prepared by or submitted by the out-of county medical examiner or someone under your direction in a manner not expressly authorized by the attorneys should be requested, notification of the Anderson's lawyers of any request by anyone to examine, inspect or copy such documents or records, or any attempt to serve or the actual service of any court order, subpoena or summons upon the Anderson's, is requested.

The forensic pathologist, retained by the Anderson's attorney, noted that since this was the third autopsy and she had not been apprised of the circumstances of Alice's death and had no knowledge of what other people's conclusions were along the way, this was a difficult situation for her. She was, for unknown reasons, unable to talk to Dr. Wyman as would be protocol in these cases. She noted that Dr. Wyman was a very stubborn and arrogant medical examiner. She also questioned Dr. Wyman's experience in pathology. Naturally she was hesitant to make any formal criticism.

A signed request from Alice's parents was enclosed as well as a deposit on any fees associated with her examination. Since state law did not require a written report of the examination, communication by telephone call was requested. There followed a request that this medical examiner's work remain confidential. This was a request to this medical examiner by the Andersons. The examiner agreed and subsequently conducted an autopsy. It revealed a Cause of Death as "Positional Asphyxia due to entrapment in bed", Contributory cerebral palsy and Accident as the manner of death. The diagnoses were: petechie of eyes, face and neck, abrasions of cheeks, nose and chin, cerebral palsy with perinatal hypoxia, seizure disorder, petit mal, and marked developmental disabilities and status post two prior autopsy examinations. The examiner knew that there was a problem with the bed and that Alice had upper torso movement such that she could move enough to cause the abrasions on her face.

The following is the verbatim report from the third pathologist:

"The decedent was a 12 year old white female with a history of cerebral palsy related to perinatal hypoxia and subsequent severe developmental disabilities including a seizure disorder that was medically controlled. She was placed in her special enclosed bed system, in the evening of 5/1/04 at 9 pm and found unresponsive in the same bed 12 hours later. CPR was attempted by the parents and continued by emergency medical personnel responding to the 911 call. She was pronounced dead in the hospital emergency room. There was purportedly no evidence of cardiac or respiratory activity upon arrival of the emergency medical team.

The autopsy examination revealed petechiae and abrasions on the face, nose and chin, indicative of compression and asphyxia. Given the circumstances, medical history and autopsy findings, the cause of death is positional asphyxia due to entrapment in bed with a significant contributory condition of cerebral palsy. The manner of death is accident.

This is a tragic accident where the decedent became physically lodged against the side of the bedding and/or rail and her breathing compromised by the compression. Unfortunately, because of the bedding and her underlying medical condition, cerebral palsy, she was unable to extricate herself and asphyxiated. Thus, the marks on the face and the petechial hemorrhages all reflect this accidental cause of death. The opinions are expressed within a reasonable degree of medical certainty."

With regard to the bed, the attorney noted that problems were generally resolved when a child could cry out or could move. With Alice, she could get her head lodged from the side position that she was in and, then, moving her upper torso she could cause the injuries to herself while asphyxiating herself.

Dr. M. B. consultation:

The medical examiner said that the tissue sections would be relevant to death by asphyxiation. The medical examiner, Dr. Wyman, did not understand how Dr. M.B. would have been able to come to a conclusion without knowing, for instance, the blood levels of Baclofen in Alice's body. Dr. M.B. had in fact been asked by the state police to review the case because they did not feel that a homicide had occurred and he had seen the autopsy photographs. Dr. Wyman did not have the bed, only pictures of it. Dr. M.B. believed that Dr. Wyman was "just plain wrong". He noted that this medical examiner had formerly been in the military and probably wouldn't change her mind. Dr. M.B. believed that Dr. Wyman was a dentist and then became a medical examiner. He believed that Dr. Wyman had very little forensic experience and made a lot of mistakes in her approach to this case. Indeed, Dr. M.B. was involved with another matter that concerned Dr. Wyman as part of a panel that criticized her opinion, so there might have been hard feelings on Dr. Wyman's part. (This case involved the death of a prison inmate. The panel disagreed with Dr. Wyman's statement of the cause of death.) Dr. M.B. eventually said that if his schedule permitted he would consider appearing in court in the matter of Alice's death.

In response to the first autopsy, the Andersons filed a complaint with the department of health involving the medical examiner's role in the investigation of Alice's death. This complaint is summed up below.

After the medical examiner and the county examiner's office took control of the case, they:

Failed to direct an investigation of the scene so that the cause and manner of death could be accurately determined. (If the cause and manner of death were not accurate, then the proper governmental agencies could not be properly notified. Without a complete investigation and careful autopsy and the accurate cause and manner of death, then the scope of interest of the health department was compromised. Homicide as the manner of death was inaccurate, causing the state police and Children's Protective Services to act upon erroneous notification by the medical examiner causing the Andersons further damage.)

Failed to examine the bed in which Alice slept.

Failed to talk to the first responders, Alice's family, her therapists or others who fully understood her limitations.

Failed to obtain Alice's complete medical history.

Failed to gain an understanding of her disability and her resulting limitations.

Failed to investigate fully other plausible explanations for the cause and manner of death.

Failed to communicate and cooperate with the lead investigating police agency.

Failed to consider two other medical examiners' opinions on the cause and manner of death.

Failed to consider relevant and complete information offered by the people who knew her limitations. (The Andersons alleged that the medical examiner failed to fulfill her statutory obligations under law and that her decision was arbitrary and capricious because she failed to consider all relevant factors. Her conclusion that a homicide had occurred exceeded her authority without having accurate, clear, complete and relevant documentation to support this conclusion.)

Failed to follow established protocols for this type of investigation.

Made a medical determination without having accurate, clear, complete and relevant medical documentation to support her conclusions.

Made an erroneous non-medical determination without justification from the other investigating agencies.

Made a faulty determination of the manner of death. (As an entirely practical matter, this inhibited the Anderson's efforts to collect Alice's life insurance as well as their ability to transfer her estate. The Andersons suffered the loss of property, expended dollars for legal defense, suffered damage against their personal and family character and reputation. This was not to mention the future ramifications including the insurance loss, loss of an estate and problems of a criminal nature. Added to this were tremendous emotional pain and distress, as well as financial burden.)

Caused an unnecessary criminal investigation and the removal of (the Anderson's) property and personal belongings.

Made an unwarranted and unfounded report to the state child abuse hotline. (This resulted in a Child Protective Services investigation requiring further legal expense.)

In a devastating critique, the Anderson's said, "Our review of the autopsy report and Dr. Wyman's conversation with our lawyers leaves us with questions. Dr. Wyman is missing important pieces of the puzzle and without these pieces we do not see how her opinion or the opinion of Dr. Sumpter can carry any weight. This case seems to be above Dr. Wyman's level of experience, expertise and education. Her confidence comes from the opinion of Dr. Sumpter. She seems to pass the whole on to Dr. Sumpter in New York. In her conversation with our lawyer, Dr. Wyman states, "I thought that maybe sending it up to New York City was really the best of all possible things . . . . you need 'premier people'". We also question the experience of Dr. Sumpter with regard to her expertise on mortality in cerebral palsy. Her opinion is held in high regard by Dr. Wyman. Dr. Sumpter wrote one report based on only 26 cases in a city with a population of 8 million people. We are hopeful when she is made aware of the details she failed to investigate, that Dr. Wyman will rethink her position and follow through with proper reporting and a careful investigation, as suggested was necessary by Dr.

Sumpter. We also trust that once Dr. Sumpter is made aware of the fact that "proper reporting and a careful investigation" was not completed in our daughter's death, she will also rethink her position.

This report by the Andersons was written while a lawsuit involving the medical examiner and her office was being considered. In the end, the suit did not proceed.

No one knew when Alice's body would be returned to her parents. Three autopsies had been performed: One by the county medical examiner, one for the district attorney's office, and one private autopsy done in an adjoining county at a well-known medical school. The last two autopsy findings were consistent with injuries previously seen in hospital beds. In addition, the state police required a review of the finding of all the autopsies. This much study of Alice's body was almost more than any of the family could stand. In the end, however, despite the local medical examiner's not paying any attention to them, the other autopsy pathologists and the consultant pathologist all agreed that her death had been an *accident*, not a *homicide*.

By now, the county medical examiner was willing to change the cause of death to "undetermined". The Andersons were warned that their estate attorney could not guarantee that the probate court and/or the life insurance company would not investigate the matter when they reviewed the death certificate. These two entities would then have to prove wrong-doing which would now be difficult for them to do. Since the certificate would read "undetermined", no charges were ever filed and there was a great deal of evidence regarding the bed. Of course, the Andersons were hoping that they would not have to deal with another investigation or other problems. They were also interested in how a cause of "undetermined" would affect their adopting a child in the United States or overseas. They wisely chose to wait further to see what issues would be raised in probate court or by the insurance company.

All this work was completed by May 8, the Saturday following Alice's death, and the Andersons began funeral arrangements. In the meantime, Millie and Robert had flown back to their Florida house, spent a day remaking moving arrangements, leaving everything else to the moving company and their friends who, to the Anderson's great relief and gratitude, even oversaw the packing and loading of the moving van. That furniture was going into storage in Florida and would be delivered to Delaware when a new house there was finished. While in Delaware they would be living in a small house they had previously built in which they spent the summer months.

So, early in the morning on the Saturday after Alice's death, the Andersons left Florida in their car. It was a long drive to Maneta, over 450 miles. They attended church in Maneta late that afternoon after checking into the motel once again. At Greg and Carol's house, cards, people and massive amounts of food were still pouring in. Greg, Carol and G3 (who was back from East Vale by then) seemed to be holding up well amidst all of this activity. One light moment occurred as they all looked around at the food baskets and other gifts of food that were stacked up in the kitchen. Even the number of people around could not have done justice to that much food.

Chapter 4

Alice's Funeral

It was the end of the week before Alice's body was finally free to be buried. By this time the Anderson's were in such emotional turmoil, they thought they could only endure one day of visiting hours. Plans were made for visiting hours to be on Monday night with the funeral on Tuesday. Visiting hours were just longer—4 hours straight. By this time, Greg's sister had moved into the house to stay with them. Robert and Millie had gone home to figure out their move and would travel back on the weekend for the funeral. Carol's parents made plans to bring G3 back at the end of the first week since the attorneys felt that it would be safe to do so.

Normal grief started to set in. Carol was sitting at the table trying to eat something when Greg's sister brought her rolling suitcase in from the car. The sound of the suitcase was like Alice's wheelchair coming over the garage threshold. Immediately, Carol had the thought "Alice is home." There was a very brief feeling of joy that suddenly turned to raw pain as the realization set in that Alice would no longer roll in the garage door. A deep gut twisting reaction occurred and Carol burst into tears and sobs. Greg and Carol eventually learned a term for the waves of grief which would seem overwhelming at times: SUG's, for Sudden Upwells of Grief.

With things quieter, Greg's sister, Carol and Greg started work on several poster boards of pictures to display at the visiting hours. As boxes of pictures were reviewed, there was one constant: Alice's great big smile. Alice had

had a happy, full and loving life. There were pictures of Alice with her brother, with her parents, grandparents, aunts and uncles and cousins. There were pictures of her at amusement parks and the beach. Pictures of birthday parties and friends. The best were the pictures of her laughing for one could almost see the joy and love of life in her expressions. Several poster boards were filled with pictures. Cards started to arrive in the mail as well. Many were filled with stories of how Alice and the Anderson family had had such a positive effect on people's lives.

When G3 finally arrived back home, Carol, Greg and G3 held each other and cried.

Carol wondered if it may have been a mistake to send G3 to her parents' house. At the time the thought was to protect him, but he also needed his mom and dad. Several years later after the death of a friend's mother, G3 and Carol had a conversation about what had happened. G3 had not understood why he went to his grandparents—he thought he was being sent away. Carol explained how scared his mother and father had been, how they were trying to protect him from more pain. She also told him how much they loved him and how "healing" he had been for their family when he was born and how he was a blessing of pure joy. G3 had spoken of feeling rejected by his parents when he needed them most. Hopefully the conversation helped him to understand what had happened.

Family and friends began to arrive over the weekend. Having people who loved Alice and the Anderson's close helped, but Carol still found herself unable to focus on the activities going on around her. There was a silver lining that Carol held onto. Her sister arrived for the funeral. Carol's sister had had some emotional problems and her relationship was strained with Carol's parents. Carol's parents and sister seemed to embrace each other in grief in spite of painful prior times. Alice seemed to have given a gift of peace as the relationship in Carol's family was and remains repaired.

The weekend prior to visiting hours, Alice's teacher called asking to bring something over that the class had prepared. These were two poster boards full of pictures of Alice at school. Greg and Carol looked at the poster and saw a child who was loved by her schoolmates. Several pictures prompted a question about Alice's being seen with the same group of girls. Alice's teacher explained that there was a group of girls who loved to interact with Alice. They were her friends and included her in their morning program, dancing, activities during field days and visited her in her classroom all the time. The teacher also had a framed picture that was to have been Alice's Mother's Day gift.

The Sunday before Alice's funeral was Mother's Day. It was a very difficult day. While out of the house the week before, Carol had seen trees blooming hot pink flowers which made her think of Alice who had liked hot pink. After a family discussion, Greg and G3 went out on Saturday to buy an apple tree to plant which bloomed hot pink flowers. It would be the basis of a garden in the backyard filled with purple and hot pink flowers. Carol tried to purchase gifts for her mother and mother-in-law, both of whom would be at the house for Mother's Day. It was very hard to do normal things. Just buying a simple gift seemed strangely to be an acknowledgment that life was moving on even though it felt to Carol as if life had stopped the morning Alice died.

Visiting hours for Alice were on Monday evening. The family arrived early to view Alice prior to closing her casket for the public hours. Carol and Greg had to decide what outfit to bury her in and a favorite comfortable sporty outfit was chosen. Along with her was her favorite talking Barncy. Carol had asked G3 and both grandmothers if they had wanted something to be buried with her. Each grandparent did have a request which was honored. G3 had expressed some hesitation to seeing his sister in the casket. No one forced him to go see her to say good bye, but just before the end of the private time he did just briefly go over to the casket. By the time visiting hours started there was already a line outside. Greg would later describe the hours of greeting friends as exhausting as running a marathon. Carol discovered that many people cared about Alice and their family which was comforting, but she also felt like she spent the entire time comforting all the visitors. The numbers of visitors never let up through the whole four hours, and she was exhausted physically and emotionally. The difficult questions were from folks who asked why there had been a delay in the services and what had caused Alice to die. When at last visiting hours were finished, everyone went back to the house where a catered meal, donated by a friend, awaited.

The funeral took place in the Lutheran Church in the village. Carol's only memory of the morning prior to the funeral was that she was shaking and all she could think about was, "How am I going to be able to do this?" To bury her beloved Alice. Several family members who had arrived later the night before came by the house. One couple in particular made Carol cry. Greg's second cousins, Jim and Maryalice, who had lost two children, (mentioned in Part I) to a genetic disease, arrived. As Carol greeted and hugged Maryalice she broke down and whispered, "How am I going to do this?" Maryalice told her she would find the strength to do it and to try to focus on people and not the actual event. The family went to the funeral home to say good-bye one last time to Alice and for a few private words of prayer from the pastor prior to going to the church. As the family left and Carol and Greg were in the car, she observed her parents and Greg's parents embrace, holding on to each other in grief. She thought to herself that it must be hard for them too—saying good-bye to a granddaughter and worried about the future of their children and grandson.

Among the pall bearers were Alice's uncle, Andy, and Alice's aunts, Joyce and Roselyn and several family friends who had known her well. Her aunt, Pat, and her uncle, Pastor Don MacDowell, were lectors. Two of her young friends, Garrett and Eric Davis, were the violinists. The music included "Humoresque", "Twinkle, Twinkle Little Star", an S. Suzuki arrangement, a violin duet, Chorus from Judas Maccabeus. The closing hymn was "On Eagle's Wings". Greg and Carol had discussed allowing family and friends to speak during the service with the pastors who indicated hesitancy because sometimes it can get long and weighty. But Carol and Greg had felt it important to allow folks to speak, and indicated that the pastors should cut it short if they felt they needed to. During the service many people stood to talk about Alice and her family. The outpouring of support and praise for such a young person and her family was overwhelming.

Robert had been sitting on the aisle just behind the other grandparents, Helga and Henry MacDowell and their daughter, Roselyn, Carol's sister. Part way through the service in the Lutheran Church, many people had risen to pay tribute to Alice. Two themes prevailed. One was the enormous quantity and the quality of love that Alice had received from her family and others who knew her. The other was Alice's sunny disposition and most especially her laugh and her radiant smile. It was plain to everyone who met her that, despite her limitations, she was a happy person.

One of the speakers was a small girl who was one of Alice's friends from school, Ellie, who was only in fifth grade. She spoke about how Alice taught her so much about love and acceptance. Alice, without words, had through her actions, gaze and smiles been a great friend. Her words were mature coming from such a young person and she showed such confidence in speaking in front of the congregation that she transfixed the crowd and stopped Carol in her tracks as she had absolutely no idea who this girl was. At that moment she seemed to be almost an angel sent from God because her words replaced the despair Carol had been feeling and replaced it with a bright sense of light.

A sudden overwhelming urge to say something overtook Robert. Since he had not given any indication that he would speak during the service, many people were surprised when he stood up, Millie to the point where she grasped her brother's hand none too gently in anticipation of what Robert might say, since she knew it had not been planned.

Without really thinking about it, Robert rose from his pew and made his way to the lectern on the side of the altar opposite the pulpit. As Robert gazed out over the congregation from the dais, two things surprised him. He was amazed to see the church all but full. And he was gratified to see so many of Alice's family members and family friends, many having traveled long distances.

Robert, "Papa", said that he agreed with all that had been said about Alice and her family, but that he needed to set the record straight on one point. "Alice did not always smile," he said. In fact, he noted, Alice was not a "morning person". Sometimes she was actually a bit grumpy after she had been waked up.

And so he told a story about Alice. It seemed that Alice did not always have her sunny smile on display. One morning while her family was visiting the senior Andersons in Florida, "Papa" found Alice in her wheel chair with a decidedly annoyed look on her face despite the fact that Barney was airing on the TV. Without hesitating, Robert placed his index finger on the tip of Alice's nose and said, in a slightly higher voice, "Beep!" With that, Alice not only began to smile, but broke out laughing. Ever after, that was her Papa's signal that all was well and that Alice should be happy.

There were smiles and a few chuckles in the church. Robert returned to his seat and the service, conducted by a young minister, proceeded until the time came for the Sign of Peace to be exchanged among the assemblage. With astonishing sensitivity, the minister announced that, for this service, all would indeed wish those around them peace, but not by shaking hands. Instead, they would all "beep" one another. And everyone did. All throughout the church one heard "beeping" going on. It seemed to evoke the essence of their dear girl and brought everyone together in mixed grief and joy.

(Robert had no way of knowing that in just a short time he would be standing in the same place participating along with Allie's other grandfather, Henry, an Eagle Scout himself, in G3's Eagle Scout Court of Honor.)

At Communion, Robert was put in mind of how tenderly Greg had broken up Alice's Communion wafer for her at Easter in Florida.

As they were in the car leaving to go to the cemetery, Carol saw Ellie, the young girl who had spoken so eloquently, and her father. She immediately opened the door and rushed over to the girl who, she had just discovered, was Alice's friend. She gave the young girl a big hug and hugged the father, telling him that he had a special daughter.

It was a beautiful mid-spring day with a slight breeze. Many of the people present in the church came to the cemetery where there was a lovely service. Caroline, Alice's six year old cousin from Delaware, who during all of this had been a perfect angel, cut balloons loose for them to rise on the breeze. The Andersons could scarcely believe all of the friends and relatives who were there from so many places. Carol was sitting in front contemplating the casket over the large hole in the earth with despair. All of sudden, a beautiful handpicked bouquet of blooming lilacs were handed to her from Ellie. Again, this beautiful girl seemed to be an angel sent from God to bring hope. Afterwards, all adjourned to the church hall for lunch.

Alice's headstone in the village cemetery is made of granite, understated. Embedded in the stone is an oval glass-covered picture of her with her famous smile. Several etchings portray Alice's life: her dog, Disco, on skis to tell about Alice's sense of humor, love of her dog as well as her interest in skiing, a horse's head for her horseback riding, ice skates and ballet shoes to remind of her other interests. Along with Alice's name are her life dates separated by not a dash but a musical note to symbolize the joyful music her life invoked. Whenever Millie and Robert are in town, they visit the cemetery.

Following the funeral life got less complicated for a brief time. At a discussion with their parents, Carol and Greg asked them to stay longer not only because of the possible repercussions from the police investigation, but because both felt so damaged emotionally from the events of the past week. Carol took one more week off from work while Greg took the rest of the week off. Both were still in shock and found it very difficult to concentrate on anything for any length of time. Carol found that gardening and working on planting "Alice's Garden" around the newly planted apple tree helped. She had never liked to garden before, but found healing and renewal as spring progressed in the gardens. Both Greg and Carol got into the habit of going over to the cemetery daily. The Anderson's had to adjust to a new normal in which everything seemed out of whack. Keeping things the same is very painful so adjustments had to be made. An example of this was the dinner table. Everyone had his or her usual spot to sit. But looking at an empty place just caused pain at every meal. So the table was turned one quarter around so that everyone was in a new place and while there is still a blank spot it is not in the same place it was. Subtle adjustments such as this occurred throughout the initial grieving period. The table is still in this turned position today.

Following the funeral, Millie and Robert moved into Greg and Carol's house. The MacDowells went home. After a short while, they returned and spent several nights in the motel. When the MacDowells returned home for good, the Andersons, Millie and Robert, remained behind to help, G3 went back to school, and Greg and Carol went back to their work. Millie went with Carol to "help out" with the water aerobics classes Carol taught. Luckily, the weather was pleasant and everyone was able to enjoy the pool.

Robert spent a good deal of time moping around being sad, depressed, frightened for his children and just plain bored. So much needed to be resolved; the legal uncertainties surrounding Alice and her family, three houses for him and Millie to deal with, not being in his own place, etc. Probably, he thought, it was the same for Millie, but she seemed to stay pretty busy. She brought lovely potted geraniums for Alice's grave and even taught G3 how to make her special garlic bread (which the Andersons have been being treated to ever since, whenever G3 is around to help with a meal).

Finally, after almost three weeks, the Anderson grandparents left for Delaware where they maintained a small home and to await the completion of their new, larger house. Except for almost colliding with a deer on the Interstate, the trip was uneventful. They were glad to be home and back in their own bed!

Greg and Carol also worked on memorials to Alice. Alice's favorite author had been Robert Munsch who wrote wonderful children's books that made you think, cry or laugh. A complete set of his books were donated to the elementary school library at Alice's school with her name in the beginning of the books. A plaque was placed outside Alice's classroom at her school that reads:

"Nicknamed "Miss Alice", "Smiley" or "Allie" to those who loved her, Alice was known for her beautiful smile that brought joy to an entire room, a sense of humor and a contagious laugh that brightened your day. Her sparkling eyes, smiles and laughter were a reflection of the joy and love in her heart that she never hesitated to share with everyone around her. Diagnosed with Cerebral Palsy at birth, Alice and her family never let her disability prevent her from experiencing life to its fullest. She was an adventurous, spirited person who was happiest when actively enjoying each day. Alice enjoyed going to school and attended Hill Elementary School. She loved roller coasters, traveling all over the eastern United States with her family to ride them. She loved sledding with her family, riding her bike around the neighborhood with her mom, going on a fast bumpy ride in her wheelchair, bouncing on trampolines and goofing around in the pool with her dad and brother in the summer. She participated in many activities including ice skating with SABAH, adaptive downhill skiing at Holiday

Valley, horseback riding at the Lothlorien Therapeutic program, bowling, swimming and dancing with Moving Miracles. She loved reading goofy stories, listening to songs by Raffi, watching Barney on TV, playing on the computer and pillow fights with her brother G3. Alice was a beautiful, bright girl whose life left an eternal impression on all who knew her by reminding us of what really matters in this world . . . . love, caring, fun, laughter and a big bowl of ice-cream."

Cards and donations had arrived in profusion and the donations were split between Alice's dance program, ice skating program and horseback riding program. An award in Alice's name was set up in both the ice skating program as well as the dance program. The extended family and friends went to the annual ice skating show later in the winter to honor and remember their beloved Alice.

In the midst of daily routines were frequent phone calls from the attorneys which upset the healing process: There was no word about the police investigation, and no death certificate yet so no word on what the medical examiner had determined. The Anderson's still did not know what had caused Alice's death.

As a surprise for Carol's Mom, Carol and Greg were supposed to be going to France to meet her parents towards the end of their trip. In a discussion with her dad, Carol indicated she could not leave G3 home and it was decided to make arrangements to take him with them. Travelling to France was very healing for the family. Carol's dad also had contrived to surprise the Andersons; when they got to their hotel they discovered Carol's sister had arrived as well. At the interment, she had felt removed and alone. The trip to France succeeded in bringing the family solidly back together again. It was the first major memory for the family without Alice.

That summer, Carol and Greg would occasionally see Ellie around town. Ellie was Alice's school friend, who had symbolized hope to Carol. A few times they arrived at the cemetery to find a handpicked bouquet of lilacs there that seemed to have been picked by a young girl but Carol did not know for sure. Alice's teacher also brought a piece of art work that Ellie had created to give to them. Carol and Greg were amazed at the sensitivity of the child. Years later, Carol was chaperoning a band trip to NYC when one of the teachers started discussing a teenage girl who had just committed suicide. Carol broke down into tears when she found out the girl was Ellie. In a twist of fate, one of the pastors who was involved in Ellie's funeral had been the pastor who had the congregation "beep" each other at Alice's funeral. Prior to Ellie's funeral, Carol reminded the pastor of the young girl who had spoken with such wisdom, compassion and sensitivity at Alice's funeral. She explained about the lilacs and how Ellie's actions had been such a gift of hope. Both shed some sad tears over how a child with so much promise could end up in such a dark place that she would take her own life. The pastor used the story at the funeral and gave Ellie's mother and grandmother a bouquet of flowers. Carol and Greg sat with Alice's teacher at the funeral and it seemed as if Alice was present as well, giving comfort to the mother of her friend—the friend who had comforted Carol and Greg at another funeral.

Personal Communications Following Alice's Funeral

Dear Carol, Greg, Greg3 and Disco,

I had the privilege of working with Alice in the classroom for a year.

All of us who knew Alice have been blessed to have her touch our lives . . . . and she was blessed to be part of a family that gave her so much love and happiness.

Love, D.W.

Dear Carol and Greg,

I will continue to cherish the time Alice spent in the class with me, especially her determination and sense of humor (She did laugh at all our silly jokes) and especially the love of family that she had. You are in my thoughts and prayers.

Love C.

Dear Greg, Carol and Greg3,

Words cannot express how sorry we are for your loss. I remember Alice at all Greg's baseball games, Cub Scouts, Sabah and school events. Her presence and her family's togetherness were very special. Please let us know if there is anything we can do.

Sincerely, K.D. and A. H.

Dear Carol, Greg and Greg3,

We think of you when we think of people who are loving and kind. We will always remember how you took Alice everywhere with you—swimming, ice-skating, skiing, Boy Scout meetings and bowling. You showed such love for her—it was always so inspirational to see you live out care, concern and striving always for a close-knit family. As parents we always saw you being selfless and generous to Alice. What a gift she was to all of us. We remember her smiling at Greg's 40th birthday party. We remember Alice's joy as the "marshal" of the Pine-Wood derby.

Please know that you are in our thoughts and prayers during this sad time in your lives. May the hope and peace of Jesus be a very real presence in your lives.

Love, G.B. S.M. T.J. and A.

Dear Anderson family—

Words cannot truly express how sorry we are for your daughter's loss. We know what a close and wonderful family you have. We have always been inspired by all you do for your family.

We are sincerely sorry and want you to know we are thinking of you

With love, M.M.K.K.L.

Carol, George, G3, grandparents—

There are really no words to express the empathy we have for you, the gratitude for the gift of Alice in our lives. The happiness you instilled in her was always evident and she did not hesitate to share her joy with everyone around her. Because of you, her life was a very content and purposeful one. You were always such a role model for us and every other family that had a child with a disability. You made sure she had the best: great teachers, fulfilling activities, laughter and fun, surrounded by those who loved and appreciated her abundant qualities—cheerfulness, sense of humor, love of people, music, animals. Her life is a reminder of how precious the gifts of our children are from God. We are comforted to know she is in Heaven, dancing, singing, riding a beautiful horse, skating, having a great time with Erica and I know her spirit will always be with us—but we will miss her so much. You are in our prayers always just as Alice will be in our hearts.

Love and God's blessing, C.B. and family.

Dear Carol, Greg and G3,

Our prayers are with you every day. God bless you in your days ahead.

Alice was so lucky to have such wonderful parents and a loving brother.

She is in Heaven and loving you each day.

Love, K and E.

We will always remember Carol holding Alice, sitting so close to her. We remember Carol and Greg feeding Alice with such love, compassion. Never any impatience, just generosity. We remember her being the marshal at the Pinewood Derby, Greg holding her in the pool on the way to Florida in '03, Carol holding Alice on a blanket at soccer games, bowling with the Boy Scouts.

You all are an inspiration to us in love. Thank you—you are in our prayers forever. Thank you Alice for teaching us to be happy.

Love, G.B.F.

Dear Alice,

Though we live far away and haven't shared as many smiles as we would have liked, you have touched our hearts and brought much joy to our world. All of your accomplishments and the love that you have brought out in your father and mother and brother have made our lives very special. Your life is always a reminder of what really matters . . . fun, love, caring and laughter.

We are grateful to have been touched by you and please know you are always in our hearts.

All our love, R.W. and S.B.

(R.W. and Greg have been best friends since they were 5 years old, going off to kindergarten together.)

Dear Alice,

We will never forget your huge smile and great laugh. You taught us so many things. You taught us to never underestimate you. Every time we saw you or talked to your mommy and daddy we learned of some new activity you had begun or some new skill you had mastered. Thanks for all the fun on roller coasters and bumpy paths, and for letting Poco lick you all over. We will miss you so much!

Love always, Uncle C., Aunt T., Caroline and Blake.

P.S. Uncle C. (a police officer) will make sure no one ever parks in your (handicapped) parking spaces.

I remember every time I think of Allie, her laugh. She had the best and most infectious laugh of all—it always made everyone in the room laugh. And her favorite was her little brother Greg3. She loved him so and loved to laugh when he came to visit us in school!

S.W.

We remember Alice's constant smile and going to one of her SABAH shows. Her smile and love touched all of our hearts.

Great Aunt and Uncle MacP.

Every time I went to G3's I was used to seeing Alice and now she isn't there and I miss her so much. Going to G3's isn't the same anymore.

M.L. (one of G3's best friends)

When we went to Alice's SABAH show this past winter, I had tears in my eyes during the entire performance. She was a shining star that day, as she worked so hard to be a part of the show.

Thank you Alice for teaching all of us about perseverance in the face of daunting challenges. I learned so much from you in the short time I knew you. You meant so much to M.L. You will be missed a great deal. I asked God to watch over you and to make an ice rink and a bike path just for you.

Love, Mrs. L. (M.L.'s mother)

Chapter 5

Conversations with Greg III

(G3 is named for his Great Grandfather, Gregory. His father is named after his Grandfather. Since a generation is skipped, Gregory III gets his title in the royal fashion. His nickname has been G3 since the beginning and he still responds happily to that designation.)

Imagine if you will, receiving a letter from the county Department of Social Services, Child Protective Services, informing you that "you are the subject of a report of suspected child abuse or maltreatment received by the State Child Abuse and Maltreatment Register. This means that you have been identified as the person(s) who is responsible for causing or allowing to be inflicted, injury, abuse or maltreatment to the child(ren). The county will commence an investigation and evaluation of the allegations in the report as required by the State Child Protective Services Act. If the report is determined to be "unfounded" it will be legally sealed." This is precisely what happened to Greg in early August 2004. Much of what follows is in reaction to this letter.

Carol's first contact with CPS was with a business card tucked into the front door asking the Andersons to call the Service. Carol was thankful that neither she nor G3 was at home when the agent came.

The Andersons did not know what was going on in the case from early May until August. Their first indication that all was not well came with the visit from the CPS agent. For three months everything was quiet but they were on pins and needles the whole time.

In early August 2004, Child Protective Services (CPS) received a report that in May, Alice had been found unresponsive. It had been determined that she died by asphyxiation and had very suspicious bruises on her face. The death had initially been ruled a homicide. The CPS agent was aware that there were conflicting reports as to the cause of Alice's death. Because of the report, she was required to assess the safety of the Anderson's home. She also wanted to interview G3 and possibly obtain some collateral information including information from care-givers, pediatricians and schools. She also requested information regarding Alice as well as her parents' version of what happened the day Alice died.

A CPS agent said that she had spoken with the state police concerning the Andersons. The police, she said, had been very complimentary of the Andersons.

The agent did not have a copy of the third autopsy. The medical examiner there had noted "innocent explanations" for what had happened to Alice.

The agent then told the Andersons and their attorney that she did not believe that the case had any merit and characterized her report in that regard as "unfounded", but that she was under pressure from her superiors to continue the case, despite her findings.

Two days later the agent called the attorney to reiterate the importance of interviewing G3 as soon as possible. By this time the agent had two autopsy reports labeling Alice's death as a homicide, one from the county and another from the doctor in New York. (Dr. Sumpter). The agent was hesitant to allow the attorney enough time to discuss such an interview with G3, but finally consented. The agent's tone at this time was characterized as "more forceful" than it had been previously.

The attorney and the agent agreed upon a date for G3's interview and would provide the ancillary information for which the agent had asked. Dr. Wyman would be invited to the interview. (She did not come.) And the autopsy report from the neighboring county would be presented. Specifically, an attempt would be made to provide innocent explanations for Alice's death. At this point no death certificate was yet on file with the county

And, so, the time came for the lawyers to talk with Alice's brother, G3, alone. CPS had asked for Alice's records, which the lawyers approved. The Andersons had been told specifically not to release any of G3's records themselves to CPS. Clearly, G3 was a smart little guy, 11 years old, doing well in school and socially well-adjusted. The lawyers prepared him to deal with people investigating the circumstances of Alice's death, advising him not to answer questions that he was not asked, not to be confrontational and the like—as one would prepare a defense witness. G3 is a fast learner.

The Anderson's attorney met with G3 at his parent's home. His report follows:

After Alice died, G3 was whisked off to the MacDowell's house arriving there without even a change of clothes, but with two books. He mainly watched TV for two days before he was returned to his parents.

When the family would visit amusement parks in Florida and elsewhere, Alice and G3 never had to wait on the usual lines to enjoy the rides. Often, the park personnel would let Alice have two rides because it was so obvious that she loved them, and G3 got to have two rides, too. After Alice was no longer with the family on these excursions, it took G3 a little while to understand why he had to now stand on line like everyone else and did not get any "special treatment". He eventually got used to the new routine, however.

G3 was scheduled to begin middle school in September. The conversation began by talking about the previous trips he has taken with his family. He told the attorney about a scheduled kayaking trip in Virginia with his mother and aunt, a family trip to France, a family trip to Florida just prior to Alice's death, as well as trips to East Vale and to Delaware to visit his grandparents, aunts and uncles. He stressed that these vacations were always family trips in which they all travelled together.

The lawyer also learned the various activities that G3 was involved in, including playing the trombone in a school band, playing soccer and baseball. He was also a Boy Scout. The theme was always the inclusion of Alice in these activities. G3 had had four different concerts in which he played the trombone, always with his father and mother and Alice cheering him on. Sometimes, when he practiced the trombone, his mother and Alice helped him to keep the beat. His father coached both soccer and baseball and his mother and Alice would come to watch his games. Alice had been chosen to be the first Grand Marshal of the Cub Scout Pinewood Derby Races, given flowers and a pin to wear. Again, G3 stressed to the lawyer that his family was always together.

G3 also had very vivid memories of Alice's activities. During these activities G3 would be present with his mother and father to support them physically and emotionally. He showed the attorney pictures of Alice involved in her various activities pinned to boards that remained in the living room from Alice's funeral.

In August 2004, the CPS agent, G3 and the Anderson's attorney met at the Anderson's house. G3 knew that the agent wanted to talk with him about what had happened to Allie. The agent told G3 that it was her job to make sure the people under the age of 18 are safe and grow up strong and healthy. The agent worked with parents to help in that process.

G3 would get emotional and cry whenever he discussed Alice. He said that he missed Alice very much and loved her very much. He described her as both a big sister and a little sister. He said that if he had a fan club its president would be Alice.

There was also a discussion with G3 about the ways that Greg and Carol would discipline him and Alice. G3 said that he occasionally gets in trouble at school mostly if he talks too much or if he forgets to tell his mother where he is going. The worst punishment he ever received was being grounded for a weekend without being allowed to play with any of his friends. He said that his parents press him to clean his room or do some household chores, but never yell or physically discipline him. He described no physical violence from his parents towards him.

Occasionally, Alice would get in trouble with his parents when she would act up at the dinner table or at other functions. Alice might yell or carry on and refuse to stop. His parents would use a "bop" to get her attention. If that didn't work, they would remove her from the table and put on a Barney video for her.

G3 said that it was sometimes difficult growing up in a home with Alice. However, he explained various ways in which his parents helped in that process. An example would be that when the family purchased their new house, designed specifically for Alice, Greg and Carol characterized the house as a "family present". The Andersons moved into this house at the time of G3's birthday. Hence, the new house became the family present.

G3 also recounted the day that Alice died. He recalled that Carol and Greg were in the kitchen preparing for breakfast while he was watching TV in the living room. His dad went to wake up Alice. Suddenly, he heard his dad in a panicked voice call for his mother. His mom quickly went to Alice's room, and he heard his mom yell, "Oh, my God". G3 said that his mom then told him to call 911 but she took the phone from him before he could do so. G3 said that he went back to Alice's room to try to do what he could to at least help out, but that his father kept him away. In the end, G3 wound up standing outside with his mother until a friend's mother picked him up.

When asked about what he did for fun, G3 announced that he swam, played soccer, and baseball and lacrosse. His dad, he said, "Is a really good coach". He also announced that he played game cube and was "a world traveler". His best subjects were science and social studies and he wanted to become a geologist because his dad is one. He said that his mom and dad were "nervous" about leaving him at home alone for longer than 15 to 30 minutes, and he wished that it could be longer.

When asked whom he would call in an emergency he said 9-1-1. "I learned that in kindergarten," said he.

He said he had his own room and the agent was welcome to see it.

Then he spoke about Alice. "Well, she was handicapped. She was nice. She had her own room. She went to school in the same district as I do, but in a different school. We would go bowling together, skiing, we would play on the computer together and we would watch movies together."

How had things changed since Alice has been gone?

G3 said, "I miss her."

He said that he has been able to talk about things with his parents, grandparents, his aunts and uncles. He said he felt safe at home. When asked if there was anything else he would like to say to the agent, G3 replied, "I went to France".

About six months after Alice died, a woman from Child Protective Services, whom G3 said he might have remembered seeing once before, arrived at G3's school. She was the same woman G3 had talked to with the lawyer and indicated that this was a follow-up on the last time they had talked. The school agreed to the visit and put G3 and the CPS worker in a room together. Incredibly, no one from the office or any of the school staff was made available to monitor this meeting. And worse, no one called G3's parents to inform them what was going on or to get their permission for the meeting. CPS told the Andersons that, legally, they could speak to G3 without his being represented. The Anderson's lawyer disagreed, but said there was little that could be done about it after the fact.

So there he was, alone with the interviewer who was on the hunt for information. No record was made of the meeting, what was said or who said what except for G3's recall.

Needless to say, Carol and Greg were at first horrified and then furious at the way this meeting was handled. Several of their friends and family advised against making a monumental fuss over it and eventually they did not. However, after a call to the school, the administration recognized that it should not have let G3 be interviewed alone, without a school representative present.

In any case, G3 informed the agent when asked that he and his mother and father were doing better now. They then went over G3's activities on the morning Alice died. She asked G3 how he thought Alice had died. He described the entrapment and the bed, since the agent had not seen the bed. (At this point, the agent and G3 had to move to another conference room which was also being used as the lost and found department. G3's comment was, "There were lots of umbrellas there.") G3 then described what activities he liked, that he played the trombone and was punished at home only by being grounded from things like going bike riding or using the computer. Near the end of the meeting, a school guidance counselor arrived to be sure that G3 was OK. Later G3 announced that he knew there should have been a "lawyer" present. He did not say anything that he thought might "get me in trouble".

In the original investigation, the CPS worker found the allegations of risk for G3 to be unfounded. It seems, however, that the agent's supervisors insisted that, because of the circumstances and the standing of the medical examiner, the agent was to change that finding and continue with proceedings against the Andersons. The family was going to the elder Andersons for Thanksgiving. Much of the trip to Delaware was taken up with phone calls to their attorney since they were now dealing with the possibility of having to go to court to prove that G3 was safe in his parent's house. The Andersons spent the month of December once again on pins and needles waiting to find out if they were going to have to go before a family court. Complicating this was the fact that the burden of proof is different in this court, and testimony in this court could be used against them in a court prosecution in criminal court. Their attorneys were concerned that some of this, such as the interview with G3, was a fishing expedition for information on the part of the prosecution.

The best Christmas present the Andersons ever received was a phone call from their attorneys two days before Christmas telling them that, based on the agent's further investigation the agent was filing an "unfounded" result. The Andersons could now relax at Christmas knowing that G3 was "safe".

When things were finally settled with CPS, the interviewer told his parents, with a degree of admiration for their son, that there had been no way at the school meeting that she was going to get any significant new information out of G3.

One of Grammy Millie's rules with all of the children was and still is "ears open, mouth shut". Saves a lot of the trouble families can get into. However, both senior Andersons carefully observed the degree of involvement with Alice's care that her parents might have expected from G3. An image of his having to form his life around Alice's needs was unsettling to Robert and Millie. Not once, however, did they detect any suggestion that G3 was to help significantly with Alice's care. G3 himself didn't remember ever being asked to help with the chores required for Alice. The younger Andersons had got that right!

G3 is now a fine, intelligent, handsome young man, and has embarked on his further education at the United States Air Force Academy in Colorado. He has many friends. Just as in his grandparent's house when his father was growing up, G3's friends all seem to congregate at his house. G3 noted that his friends all treated Alice with gentle respect. They would spontaneously slow down their activities on the trampoline if Alice was on for the ride. They would talk to her. Early on, it was hard for all of them to understand just what the trouble with Alice was, but they eventually figured things out. G3 noted that there were one or two of his crowd who were especially close to Alice. Many of G3's friends came to Alice's viewing hours at the funeral home after she died. One of them arrived dressed in a red shirt. G3 was a bit taken aback until he realized that he, too, was wearing a red polo shirt.

G3 always knew that strangers seemed nervous around Alice. These people clearly had no idea how to react to her. G3's friends were never that way, though. To them her differences were just the way things were. Carol would often invite strange children who seemed to be with their parents to come and say "Hello" to Alice. The kids usually were happy to do so and were quite friendly at the same time as the grownups were backing away, mentally and physically.

G3 also knew that, when all the legalities were settled after Alice died and his parents were "done with that", there was a sense of relief which G3 himself felt as well. He had not been paying close attention to the proceedings, but he had gotten the gist of things. Indeed, his mother and father had tried to spare him the details and they often would call the grandparents after G3 was in bed to talk about the latest developments in their strange journey.

Chapter 6

A Reenactment

Alice died on May 2, 2004. Dated May 6, 2005, was an urgent notification from the Vail bed company of improved labeling and instructional materials for several enclosed bed systems, one of which Alice had been using. It did not require owners to cease using the beds. It was noted that, "Failure to follow these instructions could increase the risk of patient entrapment and result in serious injury or death." The instructions were taken into account in the reenactment of Alice's death.

By way of the state's Freedom of Information Act, the complaint against the Vail bed company filed by the parents of a child with CP who had died of asphyxiation in her Vail bed was obtained. This suit was settled for an amount of money in excess of $75,000.00 plus interest and the cost of the suit.

The headline in one of Dr. Anderson's online medical journals, Medscape, read:

"Vail Enclosed Bed Systems Withdrawn From Market"

"June 25, 2005—The US Food and Drug Administration (FDA) has advised healthcare professionals and consumers that Vail Products, Inc., is permanently ceasing all manufacture, sale, and distribution of Vail enclosed bed systems and will no longer provide accessories, replacement parts, and retrofit kits, according to an alert sent today from Med Watch, the FDA's safety information and adverse event reporting system.

The announcement follows the agency's seizure of all finished Vail 500, 1000 and 2000 enclosed bed systems in March because of concerns that their use as recommended in the labeling was associated with a significant health risk. The FDA is aware of approximately 30 entrapments related to the use of the beds, of which at least seven resulted in death."

At the time, consumers were advised to refrain from using the devices, pending further instructions from the company. On June 23 and 24, the company sent consumers warning labels and instruction manuals that had been revised to include new warnings, precautions and instructions for use.

"The FDA advises hospitals and nursing homes to cease all use of Vail enclosed bed systems and to transfer patients to alternative beds. Consumers using the beds at home should consult with their physician about other options.

Adverse events related to the use of enclosed bed systems were to be reported to the FDA's Med Watch program by telephone, fax, online, mail. Appropriate numbers and addresses provided."

The life and times of the Delaware family who also lost a daughter to a Vail bed mirror in many ways the story of the Andersons. It is extensively described in The (Delaware) News Journal dated 11/29/2005 and is archived at <delawareonline.com>. Other beds, such as the Sorelle "Prescott" fixed sided cribs had also been implicated in young children's deaths. In this bed a space could be created where a child could become wedged, entrapped or fall. Over 400,000 cribs were recalled in 2009-2010 because of injuries and deaths of children related to the construction of the beds.

Vail did send a retrofit kit to the Andersons. There was no indication that using it immediately was a concern since it had taken the company 6 months to send the kit. Installation of the retrofit kit was no easy matter, requiring dismantling a major portion of the bed. Greg was not convinced that the retrofit would have prevented Alice's accident. Since the head of Alice's bed was raised, the retrofit would no longer have functioned as designed and required a flat-lying mattress. With the head of the bed raised and a lot of give in the netting, however, Alice could have gotten her neck caught over the bed rail and/or slipped into the space that existed between the mattress, the netting and the bed rail. Gravity would have been a factor.

In addition, the pictures the state police took of the bed while they were in the house showed the bed made with pillows neatly arranged, the large discolored spot on the netting was covered by a pillow. With relatives and friends coming to the house, the Andersons had washed the sheets and made up the bed. Two of the medical examiners would not have even seen the spot on the netting in the pictures they reviewed.

There were at least 26 new adverse events with the Vail Bed reported to the FDA by the manufacturer during the winter of 2005-2006 in which there were injuries and/or deaths. Eighteen of these events involved incidents between the mattress and side of the bed, either the bed rail or space between the bedrail and the end of the bed on the side. One of the reasons that the Andersons bought the bed was for the ability to raise the head end of the bed. The company was still selling beds to the public, not just to medical facilities. It is reasonable to expect a hospital or nursing home to "vigilantly observe and supervise patients" according to the company, but Carol wondered about home caregivers. They would be sleeping at the same time the person is using the bed and probably could not afford a nurse/aide 24/7. It would not be reasonable to expect a parent to wake up every hour or so to check a child. The Andersons went the extra mile with an intercom system so that they could hear Alice, but that would not have helped, nor would a video monitor. Even if one did check every hour, loss of oxygen leads to death within minutes. The conclusion was that the directive from the company was not helpful.

In late April 2005, the state police returned Alice's bed (which they had taken apparently to do a reconstruction and which did not happen), bedding, riding helmet, and pajamas. It was difficult for her parents to see the comforter, pillows and Allie's star pajamas, but they experienced a sense of relief that it all was back in their possession. At the Anderson's request, the police used an unmarked truck and wore no uniforms when the bed was returned. The bed was very dusty, having spent the year in a storage room. The Andersons did not examine the bed closely, but did look at the netting to discover that the staining on the netting was much larger than they had remembered and extended from the corner where the bed zipped over to the center past the end of the bed rail.

One of the Anderson's frustrations was that they felt that they were always on the defensive. When the Andersons finally got the bed back, they were able to actually support what they felt had happened to Alice. The bed contained the proof.

Allie's parents had a tough weekend with a flood of negative memories making things dark for them. Finally, on Monday, they escaped to the movies and dinner out. The next day they went to G3's band concert, plus ice cream afterward with several of their friends both parents and kids—a tradition in their group, which helped a lot.

With the idea in mind to do a reenactment, the Andersons were in contact with a Human Factors Expert with a very impressive *curriculum vitae*. He had been sent Alice's vital statistics, including mainly her medical exam measurements and weight. He also had pictures of Alice. He produced an excellent mannequin to represent Alice's body shape—Alice's clothing fit the mannequin well, and the head proportions were very close to Alice's head size and proportions.

Pictures were taken throughout the reenactment, including showing the head of Alice's bed to be a bit higher than usual because she had a cold. Importantly, Greg was able to demonstrate the position he found Alice in on the morning she died.

Since further evidence was requested, the Andersons and their attorneys decided to submit actual photos of a simulation of events in Alice's bed. So, Greg and Carol set up Alice's bed in her room, an emotionally difficult task. As soon as Alice's pillow was placed in her bed, it became immediately obvious what had occurred. The staining on Alice's pillow lined up perfectly with the vertical edge of the bed and the stains on the bedrail. There was a huge gap that a playground ball might have fit through. Carol noted that, "Our poor girl got stuck there . . . ."

Alice's bed was basically a hospital bed with padding and netting. The bed could not be pushed up flush with the wall and therefore, there were several inches between the bedrail covered in vinyl and the wall. The netting was somewhat stretchy; it had some play or "give" to it. An article from the Disabled Living Foundation (a national charity that provides free, impartial advice about all types of daily living equipment) elucidates the problem with this bed. It warns people from believing that netting and padding can eliminate areas of entrapment. It also cautioned about the height of the bedrails. In the Vail bed, netting and the wall would prevent a person from falling out of bed and over the bedrail, but, in Alice's bed, the head of the bed was angled up. When a pillow was added to this arrangement a person lying in the bed would have at least his head, neck and possibly shoulders above the bedrail.

When Alice was lying on her side, she had the ability to move her trunk forward in spinal flexion. This is the position Alice used when she had a bowel movement (there was fecal material present at autopsy). With the "give" in the netting and the couple of inches between the bedrail and the wall, space in which to become trapped could be seen. She either fell onto the bed with her neck resting on the bedrail or got her chin caught up and over the rail or possibly caught in a space between the mattress and rail. Alice usually did slip down when the head of her bed was raised. One hospital worker confirmed to Carol that it was common to have patients slip down in their beds when the head of the bed was raised, even with restraints (which Alice did not use), and commented that it was hard to get around the effects of gravity. When Greg entered Alice's room, he already knew something was wrong because Alice did not startle when he opened her door and unzipped her bed. Greg's most vivid memory was the back of her head as he reached all the way across the bed to grab her with her covers on. This meant that Alice's chin or neck was over the railing with her head twisted to the right. Two of the medical examiners involved never had the exact details of how Greg found her. (At this point, Carol wondered if the Dr. Wyman had ever seen a bedrail entrapment case.)

The reenactment went well. The Anderson's attorney, the nurse practitioner who worked in the lawyers' office and the human effects expert all came to the house. Pictures were taken using a dummy, but it was difficult to manipulate the dummy in the ways that a person moves bends, twists, etc. Finally Carol had to simulate the position of entrapment. Presumably, if what happened became clear using a 5'5" person it would also be clear for someone who was 5 inches shorter and had a much smaller head. That did work. Pictures were taken of the position she was put to bed in, the position Greg remembered Alice's being in when he found her as well as a picture taken of the entrapment. With both the dummy and Carol, there was a gap of at least 1¾-2 inches without pushing on the netting. When the netting was pushed on, the gap became large enough for Carol's head to fit into. The other interesting thing was that as Greg moved to pull the dummy toward him as he had moved Alice when he found her, his leaning on the mattress caused it to slide, closing the gap. Thus, the problem was not obvious at the time

The abrasions to the tip of Alice's nose and the bruises on her cheek had not seemed to be consistent with typical CPR rescue efforts.

Everyone was sure that this was the only explanation that accounts for everything, body marks, mucus, and liquid staining on pillow, sheets, netting, etc. The Andersons and their attorney were greatly frustrated since it was all now so obvious and no one could even get the medical examiner to discuss it. All the participants could hope now was that the pictures would be as obvious as the reenactment had been to all present. Greg and Carol recorded this as a "tough day".

In a show of respect for Papa Anderson's opinion, Greg and Carol asked him the following: First, they hypothesized that some curved marks on Allie's neck were caused by the fingers of her left hand. Second, they felt that this might be a natural instinct to reach for your neck if you are choking or asphyxiating. Allie's free arm in her bed had been her left arm which was the arm she had the most use of. They were thinking, of course, hands on one's neck would be the universal sign of choking. They wondered if this might be true, was it an instinct? They asked Dr. Anderson for his "expert" opinion.

He replied that hands at the neck do signal choking, along with a red face turning blue-purple, difficulty breathing and speaking. All but the hands at the neck are mechanical effects. This is a form of non-verbal survival communication seen in lesser primates as well, is unlearned and therefore "instinctive". This differs, for example, from the universal sign for silence—a finger placed vertically over the lips—which has to be taught outright or learned by imitation.

Chapter 7

The Death Certificate

After the District Attorney indicated that his office would not institute a criminal investigation, in part because the District Attorney's Office recognized that it would have difficulty identifying which of the three people in the house committed the supposed homicide, the Andersons continued to be uncomfortable with the absence of a death certificate. They felt that they would still be under suspicion. Two months after Alice's death, as normal grieving parents, they wondered daily what the delay was in reaching an objective medical opinion on the cause of death and determining the manner of death. They requested a time frame from the medical examiner. Maintaining a low profile as the lawyers had suggested was acceptable to them, but they did not want to jeopardize any other potential claims surrounding Alice's death. They continued to be extraordinarily angry with the treatment they had so far received from state police, sheriff and medical examiner. Among other things, they felt that they had been manipulated into being questioned without an attorney present by the state police. By this time, because of this treatment, they had already expended over $10,000 to protect themselves and their family because of what they perceived to be "incompetence and thug-like practices".

Finally, in late July 2005, the county asked Greg and Carol if they would accept a change of cause of death on Alice's death certificate from "homicide" to "undetermined".

The Andersons had always wondered whether or not an autopsy report can determine if an act was criminal homicide. Did the word "homicide" legally belong in an autopsy report? They thought, correctly, that the determination of homicide was a police function—a legal function. If the autopsy report is a medical report where injuries and cause of death are factually stated, then doesn't the manner of death have to be factually and medically supported? In Alice's case, since the state police investigation was not yet complete, didn't the determination of homicide have to wait until the police investigation is complete? Did the medical examiner step outside the scope of her job into a legal function when she leaped to "homicide" in the autopsy report without a completed investigation? Then, it became up to the Andersons and their lawyers whether or not to accept the death certificate change. This, actually, was very good news in that the medical examiner seemed determined to pursue the former designation. Her reason for doing this involved theories of her own which she was loath to depart from. Even then, however, the Andersons were still not able to access the state police forensic pathologist's report.

A hearing/settlement conference was scheduled for the following week. The Andersons were not optimistic that all could be settled with one such meeting, given how long the whole effort had taken so far.

In the meantime, the top pathologist in the country, Dr. M.B., had agreed to assist the Andersons in their case, albeit at a "really high" fee which, the Andersons thought was to be expected. If needed, then he would be able to critique the medical examiner's actions directly.

The meeting took place on August 3, 2005. Present were the Anderson's attorneys, the county attorney with the judge's law clerk mediating. Based on the information that the Andersons had filed, the medical examiner by now was "not sure what happened". She noted that she saw how the bed might have been involved, but, since the Andersons could not specifically say that when Greg went to get Alice on the morning she died, he found her head caught around the bedrail, she was unable to call her death an accident. She claimed that unless the Andersons could specifically say that they saw Alice caught on the bedrail she would not change the cause of death to "accident."

The Andersons were able to say that Greg found Alice in an area defined by the bed company as an "entrapment zone", but could not provide the specific information that the medical examiner wanted. She would not change her mind.

As has been noted previously, the medical examiner had long been convinced that deaths of individuals occurring at home were always, at least initially, to be considered homicides. This idea of hers was well known in pathology circles.

It had been clear throughout that the medical examiner didn't understand the extent of Alice's disabilities. She made statements that she did not understand how her Baclofen pump worked and why, and the correlation between her seizures and the pump. Thus, she ruled out seizures on the basis of incorrect assumptions. At this point she was still unaware of Alice's swallowing disorder. These factors would result in natural causes of death, which two forensic pathologists had already indicated was the actual cause of death. The medical examiner ruled these causes out, indicating by doing so that she felt that cerebral palsy did not play a role in Alice's death!

The meeting continued with a discussion of the issues involved in changing an autopsy report and death certificate to "undetermined" and what exactly the county was offering. The county specifically noted that it would not pay for the legal fees that the Andersons had incurred or for their emotional pain and suffering. The county specifically declined to hear an appeal because of "arbitrary, capricious, and unreasonable conduct" indicating thereby that it did not consider the medical examiner's behavior to fit this description. Also, the county was broke—out of money! Fortunately, the Andersons had been advised by their attorneys not to expect monetary damages from the resolution of a suit against the county. In the end, the county would have to get back to the attorneys about the specifics of their offer in the next few days.

Thus, once again, there would be a delay in the Anderson's decision on how to proceed; to accept the "undetermined" proposal or to make a counter proposal. They knew only that they had to protect themselves and their son, G3, for the future, and have administration of Alice's estate put exclusively in their hands. They needed the county's proposal to be acceptable on principle. They felt that they had not gone through all this to just give in. They requested a copy of the medical examiner's credentials. They also suggested that their lawyers compare the web pages in counties surrounding theirs. Their county's web pages looked to them as if they were from the dark ages of the Internet.

Three months later, the Andersons still really wanted to have the original death certificate either removed and shredded or removed and sealed. Their lawyers made this suggestion to the county, but were advised that death certificates could only be amended, not removed. Their attorneys then researched the whole issue of death certificates, county law and the Department of Health as well as state laws. They also studied adoption issues with birth certificates since the idea of doing something such as adopting had come up while Alice's death certificate was being dealt with.

Unfortunately, there were no legal means found to treat the death certificate as the Andersons desired. Indeed, statutes on the books supported the county's statement that the death certificate could only be amended. So, if the medical examiner were to change the certificate to read "accident" the word "homicide" would still be checked on the certificate, along with the words "under investigation". Later on it turned out that the town did not adequately cross out the "under investigation" wording related to the "homicide" cause of death, leading to yet more delay in the settlement.

At the request of the court, a pre-hearing conference was scheduled where their attorneys were hopeful that some negotiating might happen. No one was quite sure how much middle ground there was in the issue, but the Andersons felt strongly that they had not gone through all of this to accept any finding that still suggested suspicious circumstances as the cause of Alice's death. They still planned to stand firm and hold fast to what is true (to paraphrase 2Corinthians).

Eventually the Andersons concluded that they had proven that the medical examiner was wrong about Alice's head control issues and her capabilities. The county requested information about how exactly Alice's injuries could be explained. The Andersons and their lawyers had thought that this was the medical examiner's job. A hearing date with the county court was scheduled for August 4, 2005. The good news was that the court seemed to lean strongly in the Anderson's favor with the information it already had.

The overriding reason for the Anderson's long struggle was the principle of the matter. While there were practical financial reasons for the Andersons to fight on, they did not want the charge of "homicide" hanging over their heads. They felt they needed to have their situation reflect the truth and to have the wrongs against them corrected. They wanted the truth to be known widely so that others in similar situations not become prematurely discouraged.

Finally, though willing to have a change on the certificate to "undetermined", the Andersons were told that their estate attorney could not guarantee that the probate court and/or the life insurance company would not investigate the matter when they reviewed the death certificate. These two entities would then have to prove wrong-doing which would now be difficult for them to do since the certificate would read "undetermined". No charges were ever filed and there was a great deal of evidence regarding the bed. Of course, they were hoping that they would not have to deal with another investigation or other problems. They wisely chose to wait further to see what issues would be raised in probate court or by the insurance company or with regard to Alice's estate.

Concerning the latter: The following exchange between the Andersons and their lawyer is an example of the anxiety the Andersons were forced to live with. They wanted to be sure that they would be able to control the monies that were due to Alice's estate, and so they asked for clarification from their lawyer.

The lawyer responded that, under the state law, a person cannot profit from one's own wrongdoing and a person who would stand to inherit as a result is disqualified as an heir. Likewise, an insurance company does not have to pay benefits in like circumstances. If the issue is raised, the surrogate court would have to appoint a guardian *ad litem* to protect G3's interests since he would become the heir if his parents were disqualified. Theoretically, with "undetermined" on the death certificate, the court or the insurance company could raise the issue. G3's guardian then would be obligated to reopen the whole issue. Practically, the parties involved could not prove that there was wrongdoing and the evidence overwhelmingly shows that the design of the bed was the cause of Alice's death. In probate court, the standard of proof is the preponderance of evidence (50% plus 1%) and the burden would fall upon G3's guardian.

The lawyer could not see how wrongdoing would be established for either Carol or Greg, but if either was implicated, then the other would inherit and G3 would not be the distributee. He advised that, since they were in such a strong position, going forward with the "undetermined" death certificate would be appropriate.

Then, in October 2005, the county asked the Andersons to sign a release. They were willing to do so, but did not want to release the county from any potential lawsuits. So, the release would have to be carefully worded, which the Anderson's attorneys began working on. In addition, in order to further protect their interests, the Andersons asked the medical examiner to sign a written affidavit, sworn to, in order that later the medical examiner would be unable to become indecisive or deny what she agreed to say if she was ever called to testify. A written affidavit would impeach her credibility and the same document would help with probate and the insurance company.

Since the Andersons wished to control the exact wording of the release and the affidavit, as well as the wording of the actual autopsy report and what the death certificate would actually look like, they directed their attorneys to volunteer to write everything. They knew this would be costly, but they felt they could not count on the county and the medical examiner to do it properly and they needed these things to be correct.

At this point, Robert and Millie Anderson would see some humor in the way that their children discussed these matters. They sounded to them for all the world like lawyers. Sometimes it was hard for the elder Andersons to keep up with the jargon used in the reports. Alice's mother and father did go to great lengths to keep interested people, mainly family, up to date on the proceedings.

An example would be the information that as soon as the matters above were settled, a lawsuit was already prepared to bring against the Vail bed company. They had also directed their attorneys to look into the feasibility of a negligence lawsuit against the county and the viability of a lawsuit against the state police for a violation of their civil rights, alleging unlawful search and seizure of their house without a search warrant two days after Alice died. The last two of these possibilities had already been partially researched and, for various reasons, reached dead ends.

As part of their settlement demands, Greg and Carol asked to speak directly with the Dr. Wyman, who understandably by this time, was not thrilled with the idea. They felt that they needed to produce an understanding in the medical examiner's mind of Alice's medical issues and how they were related to her death. They also still felt that they needed answers from her as to why she acted upon the death certificate the way she did. Greg and Carol actually asked the people following this story for input on what questions should be asked. Over their protests, they had to agree to a confidentiality clause in the settlement agreement. This was at the urging of their lawyers, even though it meant that the medical examiner could testify that her first opinion was "homicide" if asked to testify by the insurance company. In contrast, it would also mean that their lawyers would have little if any room to negotiate. Greg and Carol decided to take their lawyers' advice.

Once matters were finally settled, they were planning on filing a written complaint against the medical examiner with the state. While this plan might not have legs, they were hoping for a permanent record as a way of helping other families in the future.

Then, under intense pressure from the Anderson's attorneys, Dr. Wyman agreed that subsequent to the completion of the autopsy report, and subsequent to her receipt of Dr. Sumpter's review referred to in the autopsy report, she had learned new facts, including information about the bed Alice slept in, which could have entrapped her. This new information received about the bed caused the medical examiner to change her opinion as to the manner of Alice Anderson's death. It was now her opinion that the manner of death is "undetermined". She would amend the death certificate to reflect this change.

Beyond this, she wanted it expressly understood and agreed that this was part of a settlement of a disputed and contested claim and that the settlement was not an acknowledgement of any responsibility or culpability on the part of Dr. Wyman, the county or the county medical examiner's office.

Finally, just before Christmas 2005, a settlement of the Anderson's case was recorded in the Court of Public Records. The death certificate had been amended and the autopsy report was amended also. It was suspected that another few weeks would be needed to get the Anderson's release of their claim against the county and the medical examiner. Greg and Carol were thankful for the present that they felt God had given them in time for the Christmas holidays. In the New Year, there would be a face to face meeting with the Medical Examiner.

By state law, a death certificate can only be changed or amended to correct errors. It cannot be removed and replaced. In December 2005, the medical examiner's attorney wrote agreement to the following:

1. Alice Anderson's death certificates will be amended in accordance with the death certificate to reflect the cause as "undetermined".
2. Dr. Wyman will not sign a separate affidavit, nor will she delete the last page of the autopsy report (containing the final cause of death). However, she will add the following language to the end of the autopsy report; "Since the completion of this autopsy report on or about August 3, 2004, I have learned new facts, including information about the bed Alice slept in, which could and may have entrapped her. This new information received about the bed has caused me to change my opinion as to the manner of Alice Anderson's death. It is now my opinion that the manner of death is 'Undetermined'. I will amend the death certificate to reflect this change."
3. Dr. Wyman is willing to meet with Mr. and Mrs. Anderson to discuss the events since Alice's death, at a time and place to be agreed upon once the settlement is finalized.

The Anderson's attorneys then sent a duly executed General Release and duly executed Stipulation of Discontinuance on the merits, to be held in escrow pending amendment of the death certificate and autopsy report as provided for.

Next would come the filing of all the official, amended documents with the probate court.

Finally, in January, 2006 a general release was signed by all parties which was satisfactory to the Andersons and the medical examiner, concluding that the settlement was not an acknowledgement of any responsibility or culpability on the part of the medical examiner or her office. This occurred after the Andersons were satisfied that the release was general enough to cover their concerns such as a meeting with Dr. Wyman, and would not jeopardize their other efforts involving the death certificate, such as Alice's estate.

The idea of a civil suit was abandoned after this since the county was still "broke" and a stipulation of discontinuance was agreed to by all parties.

Once that was done, the lawsuit against Vail Beds would be filed.

The lawsuit against the bed manufacturer was settled fairly quickly. One family in another state had already settled, obtaining the better portion of money available from the company. There were two suits filed before Alice's, but extenuating circumstances, such as the fact that the victims involved were adults, enabled the Andersons to obtain a greater but less than hoped for sum of money from the lawsuit. These monies were by now, from insurance that the company, then out of business, carried. After these last suits there were no funds left. Unfortunately, after paying the lawyers and settling other expenses, there was not enough money left with which to finance a charitable foundation in Alice's name, to help with the good works that so many people in her activity groups did. This was a great disappointment to the Andersons. However, The Alice Anderson Spirit Award is given each year, at her ice skating group's main activity, to the candidate chosen by the board of the organization, who makes the most "spirited" effort to participate and improve.

But then, there would be a wait of at least three weeks to be sure that the surrogate court was not going to investigate the whole matter. That Court would have to prove that both Greg and Carol were involved in Allie's death which they would likely be unable to do since the autopsy report now clearly states that Allie's bed was involved, along with the collected evidence against the conclusion of homicide.

Chapter 8

A Meeting with the Medical Examiner

After 22 months, in early March 2006, a meeting with the medical examiner was finally scheduled. Here is an email Carol sent to Allie's grandparents: "It's been a bit busy the last couple of days with our normal activities plus we have had to go back through our entire file to come up with a list of questions for the examiner. Reliving it all again has been difficult and emotional. We hope that after the meeting it will be the end of this horrible chapter and that we will have some answers to questions that have tortured us for almost two years so that we can let go of the anger and bitterness. Our biggest concern is whether we will be able to keep our cool . . . . say a prayer that we find the right words to accomplish and finish Alice's last mission here on earth. We have always felt there was a reason why her case crossed the (medical examiner's) desk."

From cerebral palsy scientific articles:

"Proper reporting and careful investigation of mortalities in CP is required for accurate certification of cause and manner of death."

"There is a high concordance between investigator and medical examiner opinion regarding manner of death, but also a need for case review and autopsies by forensic pathologists to confirm the investigator's opinion of the manner of death, determine the manner of death when the investigator selects "undetermined", and, on occasion, to refute the investigator's opinion regarding the manner of death."

Greg explained to the medical examiner that there were three things the Andersons hoped to accomplish at the meeting. They wanted to tell Dr. Wyman about their family, their daughter Alice and how her disabilities uniquely affected her. Second, they wanted to gain an understanding of the medical examiner's role when someone dies and, third, they would like to ensure that Dr. Wyman and the Andersons understood how she and they had got to this point in a tragedy involving their family.

The meeting with the medical examiner really got underway with the Andersons showing a DVD presentation of Alice and her family. With the exception of a few pictures where her adaptive equipment was obvious, Alice seemed as if she were a typical kid enjoying typical activities which was exactly what the Andersons tried to accomplish throughout Alice's life. What wasn't always obvious was the support Alice needed just to be a regular kid.

Alice was born struggling for her life. The Andersons weren't even sure she was going to make it those first few days. They prayed to God over and over to let her live. And they felt that God did answer their prayers; she did live. Perhaps that was why it was so incomprehensible to the Andersons that anyone could even think that they would hurt their daughter. It would have been, to them, like hurting a gift from God. No one who had come to know the family and who knew who and what they were could possibly believe that . . . .

From the very beginning, Alice's parents were determined to provide her and later their son with all of the resources they needed to grow up to be happy people, and to reach their full potential. They were and are a loving, close and supportive family. With their help, Alice participated in many activities which were fun for her and helped her to obtain her highest potential. They were not the kind of parents who just dropped the kids off at a program and left. They actually participated. Alice's progress may have seemed small in comparison with other kids, but she was accomplishing her goals. As Willa Cather once said, "With great love, there are always miracles". To the Andersons, Alice was proof of such miracles.

There had been no communication between the state police and Dr. Wyman, and so she did not know that the police had taken Alice's bed, and she had only seen pictures of the bed, which, the Andersons pointed out, was a very incomplete picture. She was not privy to the Anderson's conversations with the police beyond the initial statements they gave, and she did not ask about that.

Her office was not set up to do any investigating at all.

The medical examiner seemed to be focused on the marks on Alice's face that couldn't be explained. She used this to support her finding of "homicide". Without someone's actually having seen Alice entrapped in her bed, she would not say that her death was an accident.

The medical examiner's office is setup in such a way that what the medical examiner needs to determine the cause of death is different from the police department focus in their investigation.

Dr. Wyman never conversed with the other medical examiners involved about their opinions. She admitted that, in pathology, no course of investigation is started without all parties being in agreement, but with regard to other medical examiners, this is not what happens in her office. She indicated that she was aware of the other medical examiners' opinions, but she did not know what their findings were that supported their opinions or why they disagreed with her.

In this office the official death certificate would often disagree with what the police found or the district attorney discovered. The death certificate therefore merely reflected an opinion.

As the meeting continued, Dr. Wyman spent most of her time blaming the state police. What she said may have been true, but she had not bothered to inform herself of their discoveries. Also, she would not talk to the Andersons or their attorneys after she made her official determination because she held steady to the idea that there were no findings different from the two pieces of information upon which she had originally based her opinion. Carol pointed out then that a great deal of trouble could have been avoided had the meeting that day taken place during the time period immediately following Alice's death.

And then came the shocker: When asked what she might have done differently in this case, she said that she would not have taken such a case. The Andersons were flabbergasted! Her solution and what she had learned from this case was to refuse a similar one!

As the meeting ended, the Andersons, having kept their cool, said that they hoped when something challenging came along in the medical examiner's future, that she would remember Alice and dig deeper for the real facts to come up with a proper finding.

The Anderson's impression of the medical examiner was that she was wearing the medical examiner's hat which she probably shouldn't have been, that she was strictly a lab person and seemed overloaded being Chief of Pathology and Chief Medical Examiner. She seemed "burned out", a conclusion the Andersons arrived at after comments from her about trying to get people to do things. Since she would probably do only the bare minimum on future cases, it would turn out to be a good thing if she passed complicated cases on to others.

The Andersons concluded that this medical examiner lacked the spark of joy and drive in her purpose that Alice had so clearly demonstrated in her life despite all of her disabilities.

In March 2006, Carol was appointed the administrator of Alice's estate. The probate court would do no more investigating. Just ten days later, Alice's life insurance and annuity were approved and delivered. This money would become part of Alice's estate and eventually come to the Andersons.

The following weekend the second annual Alice Anderson Spirit Award would be announced at the ice show, the Andersons taking part in the ceremony. The hope was that eventually there would be sufficient funds from the Vail Bed Company insurance to set up an Anderson Family Trust Foundation, but this would have to wait for now.

Additional Notes Concerning the Death Certificate

A communication from Carol and Gregory Anderson to their primary lawyer as petitioners in a suit to have the death certificate changed so as not to include a "diagnosis" of "Homicide". The Respondents in the suit were Dr. Wyman, the county medical examiner's office and the county. Their Preliminary statement was as follows:

Petitioners have commenced this proceeding pursuant to Civil Law and Practice Rules (CPLR) Article 78, seeking a judgment granting them various forms of relief, in the nature of mandamus (command that a certain thing be done) and in the nature of certiorari (a request for a review of a record of a case). Respondents have served their Answer in which they pled their responses to the various allegations contained in the Petition, and in which they have raised various Objections in Point of Law. Respondents request that the court dismiss the Petition based upon those objections. Alternatively, Respondents request the court to dismiss the Petition upon the grounds that Petitioners have failed in their burden to establish that the determination complained of was arbitrary and capricious, or an abuse of discretion.

The Andersons wrote:

We have reviewed the county's and Dr. Wyman's Answer and Affidavit as well as the county's Memorandum of Law, both with regard to the Anderson's suit. Our analysis of these documents is presented in this Medical Memorandum. Based on our review of the response papers, it is obvious that neither the county nor Dr. Wyman understands or comprehends the basis for our Petition. As you review our comments on the respondent's papers, you will find that many of our comments have already been made clear to you. Our position remains unchanged.

Because of information we have obtained over the past two months since the Petition was filed, we can now substantiate more allegations than were listed in the Petition. Originally, the Petition challenged only Dr. Wyman's conclusion of "homicide", and assumed, based on the information available at the time, that the cause outlined in the autopsy report (asphyxiation) was correct. The information we now have adds a degree of uncertainty to our original challenge and provides room for further allegations to be made. Can we, and, more importantly, do we need to amend the Petition at some time in the future?

The Andersons also wrote as follows: We find it odd that Dr. Wyman and the county deny a whole list of allegations including some basic facts. They deny facts such as the date of Alice's birth and that we are Alice's parents. These facts, as well as others, the Respondents present as true in their Memorandum of Law.

The Respondents admit to other basic facts which relate to emergency crews at our house, pronouncement of death at the hospital and the requirement to have an autopsy. Notably, Dr. Wyman neglected to respond to the statement that she did not examine Alice's bed, did not talk to the first responders, Alice's family and those people who understood her limitations. This lack of response conveys several notions, including: they did not respond because they already knew of these facts, or they just plain forgot to respond, or they failed to comprehend the impact of Alice's disability on every aspect of her daily life.

The Respondents do admit to the importance of the medical examiner's office to the community, but deny that we, as parents, have a great stake in the medical examiner's determination. This point is further discussed in the Memorandum of Law.

We are unable to respond to certain arguments of the Responders because they are fuzzy, unsupported and/or not clearly substantiated in the Memorandum of Law.

Memorandum of Law

Our comments with regard to the Memorandum of Law are given in an *instinctual* context as we have no legal basis with which to evaluate the arguments presented.

The Respondents state "the gravamen (the essential part of a complaint or accusation) of our claim is that the autopsy report and death certificate are based on an incomplete investigation and therefore Dr. Wyman's conclusion . . . . is arbitrary, capricious and an abuse of discretion." We maintain that an equally important claim is the failure of Dr. Wyman to perform her duties as entailed by law. The Respondents appear to disregard this point.

The Respondents state that we do not have standing to bring a petition because we do not meet a two-part test. The alleged test states that:

1. We must have a legal stake and suffered actual harm because of the administrative action, and,
2. The injury must fall within the zone of interests promoted by the statutory provision under which the agency has acted.

If it is true that we must meet a two-part test, we feel we do have a legal stake in the matter, having suffered injury as a result of the medical examiner's actions. There is no need to use conjecture, the damages are obvious—we have been harmed by the medical examiner's actions. First, Dr. Wyman's reporting of the supposed homicide to the state police resulted in an unnecessary criminal investigation and the removal of our property/personal possessions (Alice's bed) from our residence. Similarly, Dr. Wyman's report to the state Child Abuse Hotline resulted in an unfounded Child Protective Services investigation. In addition, we have been forced to expend money to hire an attorney to defend our interests in both of these matters.

Dr. Wyman's reports to the state police and Child Protective Services and the resulting investigations have also damaged our reputation within the community, both verbally and in print and defamed our character. Many of the people we know in our community were spoken to about this matter including our children's teachers, counselors in school, our doctors, and the staff members of programs that our children are involved in (the therapeutic riding program, for example). In addition, our entire neighborhood watched as Alice's bed was removed from our residence by a platoon of state police. We were forced to have our son taken to Westvale by his grandparents to protect him from what seemed to be the imminent arrest of his parents. This at a time when he needed his parents both emotionally and physically.

The death certificate is a written public record. Since there is no statute of limitation on a homicide, Dr. Wyman's erroneous determination will impact us with an ever present cloud for our entire lives. In addition, the death certificate affects our efforts to collect life insurance as well as our ability to transfer Alice's estate.

We feel that we have suffered from the loss of property, have expended dollars in our defense, suffered damage against our personal and family character and reputation, not to mention the future ramifications including the loss of life insurance, an estate and future criminal problems. Add to this the tremendous emotional distress, financial burden and pain caused by this nightmare. The Respondents were apparently the only persons who believed there was a homicide. Therefore, damages incurred are a direct result of the Respondent's notification of homicide to the state police and abuse to the Child Protective Services. We definitely meet the first test.

The second part of the test involves a zone of interests that the agency has acted upon. If the Respondents are correct that the Department of Health's duties are to promote public health and inform relevant agencies of causes and manners of death, then a correct determination of the cause and manner of death is mandated. If the cause and manner of death is not accurate, then the proper governmental agencies cannot be properly notified. Notification with inaccurate information shows the Respondents failed to fulfill the duties conveyed upon them by law. Without a complete investigation and careful autopsy, the accurate cause and manner of death cannot be determined, thereby compromising the zone and/or scope of interests of the Health Department. Here, homicide as the manner of death, is incorrect. The state police and CPS acted upon the erroneous notification by the medical examiner and caused us damage as a result.

Also, it is inconceivable to believe that a parent's need to know why their child died is not part of the Health Department's zone of interests and would not give the parent a legal stake in the outcome. As parents, we have an inherent stake. The cause of death may have a direct impact on the health of other children in our house, us and our relatives. An example of this is the case of a genetic defect or a disease that presents us with risk factors to our own health. Family medical history is very important and the cause and manner of death helps to fill in these blanks. In addition, we as parents are members of the community the Health Department serves; they are obligated to fully serve us as they would any other member of the community. An incorrect determination of death promotes none of these ideals.

The Respondents state on page 4 of the Memorandum of Law that emotional distress would not be considered a legal stake in this proceeding because of a prior decision in a negligence action. Our Article 78 proceeding is not parallel to a negligence action. We are not alleging negligence at all. We are alleging that the doctor failed to perform her job as required by law and that she rendered a decision that was arbitrary and capricious. In addition, it is not just Dr. Wyman's conclusion that is painful; recent information puts her determination of the cause of death in question. The whole process from the moment the medical examiner entered the picture has caused us damage.

With regard to the assertion indicating that we are not without remedy, what other legal contexts are the Respondents referring to? If the referred to legal contexts are criminal court and family court, we would not be facing those issues if the death certificate were accurate. If the fact finder is Dr. Wyman, we point out that she has repeatedly refused to hear our point of view (facts). In addition, we have to object to the word "vindication". Our action is not about our vindication, it is about Dr. Wyman's failure to do her job—to determine our daughter's cause of death. It is about justice for Alice and about correcting an incomprehensible wrong done not only to our daughter but also to her family.

Our action is also about the rights of the disabled who, according to Dr. Wyman, deserve a "proper and thorough" autopsy and investigation just like any non-disabled person. It is about the rights of the disabled to be considered contributing members of society without a medical examiner jumping to the conclusion that a disabled person is such a burden to their family that we, as parents, would abuse and kill her (CP inconvenience). Our action is about the rights of the disabled to be viewed as equal to other non-disabled members of the community. As a family, we have been confronted with uninformed people who viewed us as "white trash" because we had a disabled daughter. The medical examiner's preexisting prejudices about disabled people being a burden to society and inferior are the spark that ignites her presumption of guilt and alters her objectivity. Perhaps we should be alleging prejudice and a violation of Alice's rights as a disabled person.

It appears the Respondents are claiming we do not have the right to direct Dr. Wyman to change her decision because we failed to state a cause of action upon which relief may be granted. We argue that we do have a legal standing to bring a cause of action. Therefore, we do have the right to request the court to direct Dr. Wyman to change the certificate. We also argue that we have clearly stated a cause of action for relief by alleging that the medical examiner failed to fulfill her statutory obligations under law and her decision was arbitrary and capricious because she failed to consider all the relevant factors. The Respondents state that her conclusion was made within her statutory obligations and that we do not claim that she has exceeded her authority. While the doctor's statutory obligation may have been fulfilled in a general sense, her conclusion of a homicide exceeds her authority by notifying the police and CPS without having accurate, clear, complete, and relevant documentation to support her conclusion.

Their argument is that Dr. Wyman's conclusion is not only discretionary but one of professional judgment. The doctor claims that her investigation was proper and thorough. The Respondents claim that the standard of review is simply, "did Dr. Wyman lack any reasonable basis for her conclusion" and that Dr. Wyman's conclusion has to be "evaluated using the same data she used". They also argue that the medical examiner's determination is not arbitrary and capricious, but has a reasonable and rational basis. Therefore, we are not entitled to have the determination annulled. If their assertion about the standard of review is correct, and that the medical examiner's conclusion has to be evaluated using the same data, we would argue that her decision is arbitrary and capricious, based on her failure to use proper discretion, failure to use reasonable professional judgment and failure to conduct a proper and thorough investigation. This is a question of fact that should be determined by the court.

Respondents state that Dr. Wyman is required to fully investigate the essential facts. They emphasized the word *essential*. We would emphasize the word *fully* and the word *facts* as well. Dr. Wyman felt the educational records were essential because she obtained them to support her determinations. However, she cannot claim she investigated the facts in the educational reports fully because she arbitrarily discounted equally objective, and, in some cases, medically supported pieces of information. A review of the records supports this assertion. Information is present in Carol's statement and the ER report challenging Dr. Wyman's statement in her affidavit that Alice was put to bed on her side and woke up on her side. She assumes that the positions are the same, yet Carol's statement indicates there was fluid on the netting, the ER report states Alice was found on her side, head into the mattress. She failed to see the questions in the data she was given that would challenge her assumptions because she was not acting objectively. In addition, how can one know if one has missed anything essential if not all of all the information is available in the case?

There must be court decisions with regard to the degree of due diligence a professional owes to his or her duties, outlined under law. Alice was a child with numerous health problems; Dr. Wyman herself admitted to our lawyer in a conversation in August that this was a difficult case. Even Dr. Sumpter indicates in her paper on CP deaths that a careful and thorough investigation is needed to determine the cause of death. Dr. Wyman is aware of all this, yet she made only a half-hearted attempt to gather information. She has provided not one recent medical recording of the material attached to her affidavit. She has provided recent educational records only. Note that these records are records we provided to the pediatrician. They are by no means the complete educational file. In essence, Dr. Wyman used educational reports to make a medical determination. This cannot be perceived as good medical or professional judgment.

In the educational report there were medical professionals she could have contacted to find out more about Alice's capabilities especially since she states in her affidavit she thought about her head control issues. She doesn't even appear to have read the complete educational report, only the first paragraph of Alice's current educational report stating her educational levels. She was not aware of so many of her health problems. These include her trunk and head control problems, her seizure history after her Baclofen pump was placed, her swallowing disorder that was, in retrospect, worsening, even her recent history of a major sinus infection. Another pathologist's report seems to lend credence to these issues being essential. A doctor in a clinical setting needs a complete medical history so as to make an accurate diagnosis and avoid complications. Dr. Wyman failed to do a very basic job. How can this be perceived as thorough? There is an expectation of due diligence on the doctor's performance of her job.

In addition, we noticed that they failed to quote the entire county law that we referenced in our Petition. They only addressed the phrase "fully investigate the essential facts concerning the death". In our view the rest of the law is pertinent since Dr. Wyman failed to take possession of Alice's bed and she admits in her affidavit she did allegedly consider positional entrapment, but failed to investigate the possibility that Alice's bed was involved.

In our response we need to make clear that this is not a "simple matter of *one* reasonable mind disagreeing with another". A lot of reasonable minds disagree with her, indicating she is just plain wrong, including three other pathologists. Is it universally accepted in this area that reasonable minds may disagree? We would hope that forensic science is more than just hypothesis up for argument. We believe that if proper scientific investigation techniques are used, all the data collected should support the conclusion.

If it is true that the standard of review is simply did Dr. Wyman lack any reasonable basis for her conclusion, and that we have to use the same data that she used, we believe her data gathering process was full of mistakes. Therefore, her conclusion cannot be considered reasonable. Since Dr. Wyman used data arbitrarily chosen to support her conclusion while arbitrarily discounting other conflicting pieces of data from the very same reports, her conclusion cannot be perceived as reasonable. She quotes the emergency room doctors' report, yet arbitrarily discounts the statement that there was no other trauma. She arbitrarily pulls out a statement from the educational reports that state Alice can lift her head when requested (written by a teacher), but arbitrarily discounts other pieces of information made by other medical professionals in the same report which state she can only hold her head in extension for 5 seconds. The occupational therapy goals in the same report state improving Alice's head control is a goal. The educational report even talks about a wheelchair with a head support. All this information in the educational report seems to challenge her conclusion that Alice had reasonable head control.

She claims that her decision is based on her knowledge, education and experience. Yet there are barometers of job qualification or minimum standards of knowledge that a Chief Medical Examiner would be expected to know and use. Her discretion cannot exist in a vacuum. There has to be external performance factors of her job. If a medical examiner's decision is solely based on knowledge, education and experience of the person in the job and the coroner is to be measured only against that, then anyone could be a medical examiner, render an opinion and say it was accurate based on their knowledge, education and experience. It sounds ridiculous when thought of that way, but isn't that what Dr. Wyman is stating? What are the criteria that a reasonable person would use to judge the accuracy of a medical examiner? What are the minimum standards of the job? It is those barometers that also have to go into the equation of determining if Dr. Wyman lacked a reasonable basis for her conclusion and used her discretion correctly. If she failed to follow and meet the minimum standards, then Dr. Wyman failed to perform her duties entailed by law.

It is the preponderance of all this information which tips the scale in our favor on arbitrary and capricious. Definitions of arbitrary and capricious we found state that it is: 1. The "absence of a rational connection between the facts found and the choices made" and 2. "A clear error of judgment; an action *not* based on the consideration of relevant factors and so is arbitrary, capricious, an abuse of discretion or otherwise not in accordance with the law or if it was taken without observance of procedure required by law." In the first definition, if one arbitrarily discounts some facts, fails to fully collect all the facts and erroneously makes assumptions, we can say there was not a rational connection between them. In the second definition, we would assume a reasonable person would look at all the facts and relevant factors and follow established protocols and minimum standards as well as be objective. A failure to follow a minimum of standards, a failure to follow the established protocols of the job, a failure to consider relevant factors and possibly adding in preexisting prejudices involving people with disabilities has to be seen as a clear error of judgment, not reasonable, and therefore arbitrary and capricious.

In the Memorandum, Respondents state Petitioners only disagree with the conclusion of homicide. Aren't we in fact now arguing that we not only disagree with Dr. Wyman's conclusion, but disagree with the entire process she used to supposedly do her job? We disagree with her judgment and her discretion. We now have strong information that the data evaluated by Dr. Wyman is erroneous, suspect and simply not true. We know she arbitrarily picked out certain pieces of data while ignoring other equally objective and believable pieces of information. Aren't we in fact challenging her qualifications to be a chief medical examiner? We have been asking ourselves why she was hired to be a chief medical examiner without a certain prerequisite level of skill and experience in forensic science. Should our Petition be alleging these issues against the county? In the very least, such allegations involve Dr. Wyman's supervisors/managers in this lawsuit. Pressure from these sources may be what is needed to effect a change in Dr. Wyman's attitude.

Finally, we find it very important that the Respondents do not argue against our right to ask the court to direct Dr. Wyman to investigate the death fully. Aside from issues of legal standing, this is the one form of relief we have requested from the court which the Respondents have not challenged. We are worried that the court will in fact grant this form of relief and we will be left with an investigation completed by an individual who is complying against her wishes, belief and under duress and therefore not even close to objective. Is there a way to work into our response or in an amended Petition a request that an independent third party medical examiner complete the investigation at the Respondents' expense?

A Rebuttal of the Affidavit of the Medical Examiner

Paragraph 1. In which Dr. Wyman lists her credentials and says that she is personally familiar with the facts set forth except those matters as stated to be upon information and belief, but as to those matters she believed them to be true.

The Andersons note that Dr. Wyman fails to supply the number of years of experience she has in forensic science. Dr. Wyman asserts lots of certifications and education, but what about on the job experience as a forensic pathologist?

Paragraph 2. Here, Dr. Wyman says that when she first viewed Alice's body, she noted various markings on her body, as a result of which she requested that representatives of the investigating police agency attend the autopsy.

The Andersons note that Alice apparently was not viewed by Dr. Wyman until day 2 after her death. Was she investigating markings on the body and their source, or a predetermined cause/manner of death? We believe she had already formed an opinion of homicide based on the markings which was conveyed to the police. We would want to know what exactly she said when she notified the police agencies.

Paragraph 3. Dr. Wyman reviewed written statements given by the Andersons to the state police Investigators.

With regard to our statements, our feeling is that Greg's statement lacks important details about the exact position Alice is found in. This is important because it is not the same position in which Carol put her to bed.

Paragraph 4. Dr. Wyman says that Alice was placed on her right side in the evening and was found on her right side and unresponsive in the morning.

She also says that, according to hospital records which she reviewed, Alice had been deceased with cardiac arrest "at some point through the night".

It is important to note that Carol was the last to see Alice in bed in the evening, while Greg found Alice in the morning. Dr. Wyman is making the assumption that Alice went to bed in the position she was found in, in the morning. That detail is not clear and should have caused Dr. Wyman to ask for the exact positions. Dr. Wyman states she reviewed both of our written statements, but she only refers to "Mr. Anderson's" words. She quotes the hospital report as stating cardiac arrest as the cause of death. Again, as we have previously indicated, on the morning of Alice's death, what we observed in her bed looked more like a positional problem. That belief is reflected in the emergency room statement that we found Alice "on her side face down into the mattress". No one asked us for any details including the state police or the sheriff's department on that day.

Dr. Wyman does not respond to our note that she never examined the bed in which Alice died. Likewise, she never spoke with those who understood most about Alice's cerebral palsy and her limited movements, the individuals who last saw her alive, the individuals who tried to save her life, or her family. But, she admits that she did not talk to the first responders. She formulated an opinion only based on the hospital report in which there is no extensive description of the resuscitation effort. She only relied on the hospital report that states "no other trauma beyond an abrasion to Alice's nose and chin". While the ambulance report is present, no report is present from the first responders.

Paragraph 5. The autopsy did not take place until 2 days after her death. Alice was pronounced dead at approximately 9:30 am on May 2. Why did it take 48 hours to complete an autopsy? What happened to Alice while in the possession of the medical examiner for these two days? Could her body have been marked up? Could some of these marks have happened during CPR, while in transit in the ambulance or in the emergency room? We again point out there were no marks on her while she was in our house. Why did the police investigators attend the autopsy? Their attendance suggests that there was already a notion that a "homicide" had occurred. Who attended the autopsy and where is their report? The fact that the first responder report and investigative agencies report is missing shows a lack of "proper and thorough investigation" on Dr. Wyman's part. Did Dr. Wyman actually have the police reports to review?

Paragraph 6. Wherein Dr. Wyman notes methods used in the autopsy, concluding that there was evidence of asphyxial injury. Thus, her determination of asphyxia and her opinion that, based upon a reasonable degree of medical certainty, the cause of death was Asphyxia due to Compression of the Neck and that the manner of death was Homicide.

An evaluation of the autopsy, slides, etc. will have to come from our forensic experts, but we point out she concluded the injury from asphyxia was due to a homicide, yet has no supporting evidence listed as to why she feels it is a homicide. The microscopic exam data are consistent with the gross exam data according to Dr. Wyman. However, her conclusions drawn from a preconceived opinion are based only on her gross exam data. In our opinion, the conclusions drawn in the autopsy must consider both sets of data completely. If she didn't examine the bed, talk to first responders, completely interview us, interview the therapists who worked with Alice daily and knew her limitations, collect all the state police and medical examiner records and then consider all the data there is no basis upon which to determine asphyxia and homicide.

She lists proof of asphyxia, but gives not one detail as to what could have caused the compression, how it was done, etc. She does not look for any other reasons as to how the compression could have occurred. She also appears to discount an emergency room doctor's report that talks about the two marks on Alice's face that we also noticed in the emergency room, but clearly states, "There is no other evidence of trauma." If the marks on Allie's neck were present because of a homicide that occurred in our house, why didn't anyone notice the marks in our house, in the ambulance or in the ER?

We did not see the marks on her neck in the Emergency Room and we spent a significant amount of time saying good-by to Alice. Dr. Wyman fails to address this huge question.

Paragraph 7. In this Paragraph, Dr. Wyman very clearly shows her lack of knowledge of cerebral palsy (CP). CP is a classification for a wide range of disabilities from mild to profoundly severe. The extent of disability uniquely affects each individual. It is a disability that affects the muscle control of the entire body. One cannot just look at head and neck control in a vacuum. In many cases, including Alice's situation, muscle function is controlled by primitive reflexes. When she was upset, tired or ill, she would have more difficulty working around those reflexes to functionally use her muscles. If Alice got her head caught over the side of the mattress, bedrail or in a detrimental position, in order to free herself she would have needed more than just the ability to lift and turn her head. She would have needed trunk control as well as control of her arms. Control of her trunk, head and extremities was limited; she suffered from severe quadriplegia. She would also have to know *intellectually* that she was in danger so as to attempt to free herself.

Alice's head, neck and trunk control were affected by many factors including her positioning, her tone, how tired she was, her health and her emotional state. Her tone could change from day to day or even within the same day from morning to evening. When her tone was lower, when her extremities were properly supported, when she was well rested and not upset, her head control was such that we were looking at the purchase of a wheelchair she could propel using controls on the head support. She was still learning how to use her head to accomplish this goal and was by no means even consistent in her ability to use her head in this way. Her individual education program or IEP which was given to Dr. Wyman reflected these goals. Yes, Alice could hold up her head and lift it when asked while sitting upright strapped into her wheelchair at the waist and chest, with her extremities and trunk supported, but could not hold it in perfect alignment for any length of time.

When Alice was tired or sick, we often had to remind her to lift her head. To feed her, it was often necessary to hold her head up because she had difficulty coordinating head control and swallowing. This point is reflected in the educational reports. If Alice was lying supine, she could lift her head up only an inch or two for a short period of time. She had a self-help goal to lift her head in this position while getting her diaper changed so a pillow could be placed under her head. If she was prone, it was very difficult for her to lift up her head in extension. One would have to place her arms in position with her elbows under her shoulders and position her forearms so she could push up and lift her head. She could only maintain this for a very short period of time and it required a lot of assistance. The video from Alice's dance recital shows this.

While on her side we never saw her lift her head on her own. When in bed lying on her side, she would slide her head forward using trunk flexion. It was more difficult to do trunk extension and we do not recall that we ever saw her do extension when lying down on her side after she had her Baclofen pump placed. The pump eliminated the trunk and head extensor tone she had been using to control her trunk and her head. The educational reports support this where the teacher uses a very measureable description that Alice "can only hold her head against a switch placed behind her head in extension for 5 seconds".

Alice would go every few months to have her Baclofen pump refilled and the dosage increased. Typically, this increase is done at 10% intervals, but we found that if we increased the dosage by that much, she would have difficulty with her head, trunk and swallowing control. Because of her problems with muscle control, we were titrating up her Baclofen doses slowly at 5% intervals which gave Alice the chance to more slowly learn to control her muscles without the high tone. I believe the neurosurgery visit notes which the nurse practitioner wrote would support our reasons for slower dosage changes.

Also, Alice's wheelchair had a tilt in space option that enabled us to tilt her seating position so that we could use gravity to assist her in her head control. Dr. Wyman had photos of her wheelchair that clearly show this.

Why would she need a head support if her head control was good? She uses the term reasonable to describe head control—that is not a medical term. Head control should be measured clinically.

The pictures Dr. Wyman refers to that show her as exhibiting good head control are almost laughable. In both, she is looking down, not because she wanted to but because this was the problem with her head control. She had trouble holding her head up and this downward position was often her normal anatomical position when her body was not properly supported, when she was tired, etc. In the pictures of Alice on a horse, two side-walkers are literally holding her upright on the horse using a lot of muscle power. It was hard work. We often had to do it in her weekly lesson and the side walkers would have to switch sides or switch people because it was so difficult. She was taking horseback riding lessons to help improve her head and trunk control.

In the pool picture, G3 is directly behind her literally holding her upright on three noodles. It was not just a "flotation device". Three noodles were the minimum support we needed to help us hold Alice up in the pool. We had to use several noodles to enable her to float and we had to stabilize her trunk while swimming with her. Even with all of that, she would tire and after a while her head would sag forward.

The final picture is of Alice at her last SABAH show. She is not even looking at the camera and her head is again slightly tilted forward. The gentleman in the picture may be a good resource/witness for us. S.O., a professor in physical therapy, was Alice's teacher at ice skating for a number of years.

In addition, Alice lacked the ability to recognize a dangerous situation. If her head had fallen over the side of her bed, based on previous instances with a portable bed rail, she would not have realized the danger or even that this position was not where her head or body should be. There were numerous times she would fall over from the trunk to her side when sitting in her floor chair while watching TV and she would just watch the TV and tip over. She wouldn't cry or even make any attempt to straighten herself up. Most likely she would laugh, thinking it was funny. Dr. Wyman fails to realize that her mental function needed to be considered as well. A thorough investigation of Alice's medical problems as well as talking to the individuals who worked with her would have stricken her assumption of head control and given her a better picture of her capabilities.

Dr. Wyman's failure to fully investigate and access Alice's head control issues to any degree of medical certainty is also demonstrated by her failure to discuss Alice's head control issues with Alice's primary physician. If Dr. Wyman considered head control to be a significant issue, one that needed to be determined with medical certainty, it is reasonable to assume that she would have discussed the issue with the pediatrician and requested the medical records that define the issue. The records of Dr. Wyman's conversation with the pediatrician do not indicate that the issue was discussed. If it had been, the physician would have referred Dr. Wyman to Alice's OT and PT, as he did when the state police asked about this issue. We should consider taking a statement from the pediatrician concerning what was discussed regarding the issue of head control.

Dr. Wyman indicates that her attempt to satisfy medical certainty of head control with regard to a positional asphyxiation was "notwithstanding the marks on her body and evidence of hemorrhage". Dr. Wyman failed to recognize that the marks on her body point to the idea that she could have caused this injury to herself due to entrapment in the bed, partially because she did not understand Alice's disability and made no attempt to understand it. We were able to document the same injuries in cases of bed rail and bed entrapment on the Internet. As a medical professional, Dr. Wyman should have been aware (or made herself so) of the problems with hospital beds and entrapment. We also want to point out that Alice's pediatricians had no current information about her in their file to send to Dr. Wyman. We know this because all of the material attached to the affidavit from the pediatricians is information we gave to them after we were called to send current information to Dr. Wyman. The information is neither her medical records nor her complete educational records. It is her individual education plan. The pediatrician was not the best source of information about Alice since his records were not up-to-date. And, if Dr. Wyman wanted her medical records why didn't she contact the school district or BOCES? No medical records from the pediatricians were included with the affidavit.

With regard to these issues outlined for this Paragraph, we believe statements will be needed from Alice's teacher, physical therapist, occupational therapist as well as the therapeutic center and possibly the neurosurgical nurse or just her records. A statement from Carol about the previous problems we had with the portable bed rail as well as her trunk control issues will be helpful.

Paragraph 8. In this Paragraph, Dr. Wyman states that she wanted to know if there was any evidence of a positional entrapment.

If you want to know about the evidence, then go look at the evidence in person. Photographs of the bed do not adequately show the dangers of the bed. You cannot see entrapment zones from photos. You can't even see if a space existed between the mattress and the rail, or bed and the wall. You can't tell that the netting has tremendous "give" to it, or that the bedrail jiggles. But clues are present in these photos; they show that we were able to place stuffed animals between the end of the mattress and the bed frame. Also, who made Dr. Wyman an expert on bed safety? In order to know if any zones of entrapment existed she would have to know what those zones were. The stuffed animals between the mattress and the vinyl frame of the bed would have been one danger zone and there is obviously a gap there. What about finding out the brand name of the bed and checking the FDA web site? Or even the consumer protection agency site with the words hospital beds? She would have hit a jackpot of information. It was how we found out there were previous problems. How many years of education does Dr. Wyman have? In today's day and age we can't imagine not using the Internet for information. She even could have done research on issues involving CP, seizures, the Baclofen pump. Can we attach some of the problems we found out about the Vail beds and the FDA as well as the prior deaths, in our response?

The ER report clearly states that Alice was found on her side, "face down into the mattress". Carol's statement clearly says there was fluid on the netting and on the mattress. The medical examiner has pictures of that same stain on the netting. She seems to have simply dismissed these points. No one asked Greg specific details on how he found his daughter. The medical examiner assumes she is in the same position when she is put to sleep and when Greg found her. What parent would put their child to sleep pushed up against the netting and head down into the mattress? Her objectivity was so lacking she failed to see this as a discrepancy to her theory. She did have information that the position Alice was put to bed in is different from how she was found. She apparently discounted it or never followed up on it further. The state police took the bed, why didn't she examine it?

We also noticed that, under History in the Emergency Room report, the sentence "She has dependent lividity and bilateral corneas are cloudy." is underlined. Under Physical Examination the word "rigid" is underlined and the sentence "There is a small abrasion over the nose and chin." is circled. Since Dr. Wyman obviously obtained these reports we would assume she did the underlining and circling. These writings are reminiscent of the circles and underlines that were found on Carol's statement. This may be a clear indication of the facts Dr. Wyman selected to fit her theory. Yet, she missed the very next sentence under the heading Physical Examination which challenges her theory stating "no other evidence of trauma". Where did the trauma to Alice's neck come from?

In one of the pictures the state police took on Monday night, April 3, Carol had removed the decorative pillow from covering where the stain was on the netting and placed Alice's pillow in the position it was in on the night she died. When Carol moved the pillowcase into position, she noticed that the bottom left corner of the pillowcase had a stain on it. That would be the corner that was closest to the wall. Note should have been taken of the location of the end of the bedrail. If Alice's head was in the center, left side of the pillow looking toward the wall her head could very easily have fallen forward into the space that existed between the end of the bedrail, the edge of the mattress and the wall. The injuries to her neck actually support this as a possibility. Remember, she had fallen out of bed in this exact same gap when we were using a Fisher-Price bedrail at Carol's parent's house the prior summer. Greg and Carol both felt that the bedrails on Carol's friend's bed were longer than on our bed when we conducted our "reenactment".

There is also still the possibility of a gap between the mattress and the bedrail. We both performed CPR on Alice while she was in the bed. Our leaning on the mattress and the bed could have pushed the mattress back in place with the anxiety of the moment, and with the blankets on the bed, we may not have noticed that such a gap was there. Again, you would need the bed to determine if this was indeed a possibility.

If Dr. Wyman really thought about the bed and entrapment as a possibility, why didn't the state police ask us one question about entrapment in the safety bed? Remember, we had a retrofit sitting in our basement. We had received a letter indicating a problem of entrapment existed with the bed. If the police had asked this question, we would have mentioned the retrofit and the letter from the company to them. It was one of the first things we mentioned to our lawyer in his car while he was at our house on May 4. We were never even told what the medical examiner thought she had died of, so we didn't know if it was even relevant to volunteer the information about the retrofit kit. We don't believe Dr. Wyman seriously even considered an entrapment issue.

What other notes, verbal reports and written references would a medical examiner complete while working on a case? Are we entitled to this in discovery? If so, we wonder if there is any mention of positional asphyxiation in these notes.

Paragraph 9. As Dr. Wyman was permitted to do so by law, she requested another medical examiner, Dr. B. Sumpter, MD, PhD in a large metropolitan Examiner's Office.

Dr. Wyman sends her compromised and incomplete information to Dr. Sumpter who apparently fails to recognize the problems as well. We would question her actual familiarity with the case as she confuses Alice's name with Carol's in her letter. We note that in Dr. Wyman's referral letter to Dr. Sumpter, it appears that Dr. Wyman signs her name as "Jan Wyman". We believe she signed the death certificate with Janet Wyman. Her signature of "Jan" would indicate some degree of familiarity between Dr. Sumpter and herself and the possibility of prior conversations between the two about this case. How objective can Dr. Sumpter be if she is an acquaintance/ friend and already knows Dr. Wyman's beliefs about the case?

Also, we would not consider Dr. Sumpter an expert on CP based on one paper written which evaluated only 25 cases of CP. Such a review does not make one an expert. Does she really "concentrate in the area of evaluating decedents with an underlying diagnosis of cerebral palsy"? If Dr. Sumpter had a specialty in CP decedents, why didn't she ask for all the information?

Anyone with unbiased knowledge about cerebral palsy knows that CP is a general term that defines various classes/levels of disability. Within each class, each "case" has high degree of individuality. In any case, her paper actually supports our point about the lack of a "careful and complete investigation".

Paragraph 10. Dr. Wyman notes that other medical examinations are not part of the petitions and not otherwise identified. She does know that two other examinations concluded that Alice's death was not a homicide.

At a minimum, Dr. Wyman knows that the county medical examiner performed an autopsy in her office, and the state police consulted with Dr. M.B. during their investigation. She should have requested the autopsy report from Dr. Smith and reviewed the state police reports before reaching her conclusions. If Dr. Wyman had requested the reports from Dr. Smith and the state police, she would have been aware of the fact that there were two other medical examiners' opinions on the case. By not requesting these reports, Dr. Wyman demonstrates her failure to complete the duties conveyed upon her by law, her failure and unwillingness to complete a proper and thorough investigation, and the arbitrary and capricious nature by which she completed her obligation.

Paragraph 11. Dr. Wyman is aware that a medical examiner from a neighboring county performed a second autopsy and reviewed Alice's file. She had had no contact with this examiner.

If Dr. Wyman was aware that a medical examiner from another county did a second autopsy, why didn't she make an attempt to find out what that medical examiner thought? In a conversation Dr. Wyman had with our attorney, she very definitely was aware of the other pathologists' opinions because she discusses them with the lawyer and tells him she doesn't see what the other pathologists saw. Dr. Wyman knew other opinions existed; she failed to consider them. She can't just ignore information that doesn't agree with her opinion. Also, she wrote her autopsy report and completed the death certificate prior to receiving the written report from Dr. Smith.

Paragraph 12. Dr. Wyman maintains that her conclusion was reached with a reasonable degree of medical certainty. She notes that Alice's death was very tragic and the finding of homicide would be very disappointing and discouraging to her parents.

This entire paragraph angers us. Alice's death was tragic and made more tragic by the medical examiner's failures. It is not merely "disappointing and discouraging". What an awful choice of words for a decision that has created a nightmare out of a tragedy. We do not believe Dr. Wyman was objective, we know she did not take into account all the available reliable information and we challenge her experience and how she used her education to reach her conclusion. Because she missed so much data, her conclusion is not based on a reasonable degree of medical certainty.

We also note that she never addresses the multiple times we and our lawyers have tried to contact her to give her the information she missed. She offers no explanation for not allowing us to provide her with this information.

Apparently, she received a report on the Baclofen pump from Dr. Lee. We wish to point out that the evaluation for Alice's surgery and her surgery was performed by a different doctor and all the pump refills and follow up care were handled by the neurosurgical nurse practitioner. Dr. Lee had no direct knowledge of Alice's head and trunk control issues nor was he familiar with Alice.

Chapter 9

Going Public

There was a reporter who worked for the newspaper in The City, a friend of the Anderson's attorneys. He came to interview the Andersons in May. The Andersons felt that this newspaperman was the only one they could trust to tell Alice's story adequately and correctly. His article about Greg and Carol was a masterpiece of complete and compassionate reporting. It elicited several comments: "Too bad all parents aren't treated with the same compassion", "Innocent until proven guilty", "Without the resources to defend themselves against a rush to judgment, many are serving prison terms." "The necessity for search warrants should go without question."

"Never talk to the police without your lawyer present. The same goes for spot interviews with anyone involved."

"No doctor, including a medical examiner, is right 100% of the time."

And questions about how other parents should go about identifying the beds they were using for their children.

A television reporter whose son had been Alice's ice skating volunteer along with Carol came to the Anderson's house and did an interview that aired on the news.

Epilogue

Life proceeds in interesting ways.

One result of Alice's death ended in a difficult situation for the Anderson's extended family. The problem lasted three years and caused hard feelings among family members. The Andersons refuse now to even discuss the problem; it has been resolved to the satisfaction of all concerned and has not left any significant scars.

For quite some time, Carol's sister Roselyn and her family, Helga and Harry MacDowell had been estranged. The Andersons knew it was upsetting for Carol and her parents, but they never knew the details and didn't pry. (As has been noted, "ears open and mouth shut" is one of Millie's rules to live by.) After Allie's death, however, tensions among these individuals began to lessen. Now, several years later, all appears to be going well with the family's getting together often and allowing G3 to get to know his aunt Roselyn.

So, while one family experienced unforeseen difficulties, another family had a resolution of some problems. Overall, eventually, the Andersons were quite pleased with the results.

Not long ago, five years after losing Alice, the Andersons, Robert and Millie, attended the calling hours before the funeral of an eight year old boy. They were both fairly composed until they reached the parents with the boy's paternal grandmother standing nearby. They had never met this woman before, but all it took for them both to shed a tear was the realization that they had been through what she was going through just then. And they thought afterward that, no matter how much one has seemed to have removed oneself from the grief, to have the grief under control, certain situations evoke a tearful response. The reason was clear in this case, but during the normal course of life other situations will occur to produce the same result.

After many years, when Greg had an opportunity to work for the most part out of his house, he was able to convert Alice's bedroom into an attractive and highly functional office for himself, and, most importantly to be comfortable in it. It is an official office and very official looking with everything he needs around him to conduct his business as a manager for a large, international engineering firm in The City.

One of the items on his office wall is a beautiful wall hanging, a quilt which his mother, Millie, made out of many of the bright scarves that Alice had worn. Robert even recognized some of them. A beautiful yet appropriately understated remembrance of Allie.

Since Millie is an expert quilter, she got the idea to make a quilt for G3 just as she had been making for her other grandchildren. Robert still has the quilt his grandmother made for him in his early teens out of the dress material in which the feed for the farm animals was bagged. The farm women traded the materials until they accumulated enough material to make clothes for themselves and the family. To this day, Robert remembers some of the dresses his grandmother and cousins wore which were made out of the feed bag material. So, Millie decided to use the remainder of Alice's bandanas for the quilt. A problem; Allie's scarves were often pink, yellow, pale blue—girlish colors to match her outfits—not appropriate for a boy's quilt. Finally, Carol and Millie were able to produce a great number of bandanas containing colors that were appropriate and Millie produced another beautiful quilt for G3's bed. Beiges, browns and greens predominate. Many years later G3 is still using the quilt for his bed at home—it's probably not "regulation" as he continues his studies at the U.S. Air Force Academy.

After she had to quit her job to care for Alice, Carol became active in the fitness business. This had always been a passion for her and she kept her body in excellent shape. She began working part-time for her town's water fitness program as well as its Pilates program. Eventually she also opened her own studio in the house as a personal trainer for private clients. Her business went well, but she did not see male clients at home. When Greg began working at home, Carol was able to begin seeing male clients as well and her business grew some more. Now she has a large, modern facility at home as well as being in increasing demand in town employment as a physical trainer, often working with clients who have medical issues. So she is a very busy lady.

After Alice died and all the legal hurtles had been dealt with, Robert and Millie told some of their best friends all about what Allie's family had been through. Only a very few knew the details and the Andersons decided now to fill in the blanks for some others. Here are few of the responses they received to Allie's story. All of these people had watched Greg and his siblings grow up and knew him well.

From the "C"s: "Thank you so much for sharing the information and articles concerning your beloved Alice and her fantastic parents—They obviously went through much hell during the past four years. The conclusion shows what determination and faith can do—especially when they knew that all they did was to insure that Alice had the best care and exposure to activities that would enhance her quality of life. We know that you are extremely proud of Greg and Carol and also relieved that these past horrifying years have reached a positive end. We are also glad that the lawsuits are over and that you both can finally experience some peace of mind. We know that this experience has been very distressing for you and your family. Prayers and love to all, R & M"

From the "A"s: "Thanks for including us in the distribution of the news about Alice, Greg and family. It has taken a long and, I'm sure, frustrating time finally to get the facts in the public eye. We're sure no one really appreciates what the family has gone through. You would have to be part of it as you and Millie were to understand the tragic situation and the follow-on horror story about how the police and others reacted, with their insensitivity, unprofessional and hurtful actions. We only hope that those who are guilty get their due punishment in the public press and also personally."

"The Anderson family should all be proud of the way Greg et.al. handled the situation and their dedication to fight for what was right and truthful. Maybe the fight will not have been in vain for the family and for other families that have or may experience the same type of tragedy.

We look forward to seeing you guys this summer on the Cape." (N & A)

From the "U"s: "We were very impressed with Greg and Carol's interview/ article in the (The City) news. What an incredible amount of pressure they have had to endure. The good part is they have handled it all so maturely and professionally while keeping emotions pretty much intact. It's a chapter you will be glad to see some closure to." Love, E & D.

Alice's uncle, Robert, Jr. wrote: Cousin Benjamin remembered best having ice cream—a favorite of his—at Grammy's with Alice, and all the fuss we made. His sister Meghan remembered wearing the matching sailor dresses, ones that Grammy had made for her third birthday about the time Allie was one year old. Meghan later recorded her voice for Alice to hear at home. He wrote, "Both Benjamin and Meghan have been touched by Allie and they are truly better people for it". Robert, Jr. and Marie cherished the day spent at the water park in Myrtle Beach—the smiles and the fun on the water slide and in the wave pool with Allie. She trusted everyone. She never seemed to tire out, but everyone else did! All of us will always thank God He brought Alice into our lives. Even in this time of sadness we know she made us all better people.

The experience of Alice's death led Millie to become an active member of the Ministry of Caring, Lazarus Committee, at church. Her work for the group was recently acknowledged publically, in particular for her embroidery skills in making aprons for the Committee workers. She became a Eucharistic Minister as well at church and in the hospital.

When the Anderson's new house was completed and they had moved in they had the idea to use the front door garden in memory of Alice. Surrounded by carefully tended shrubbery, a fountain sits in the area, shaped like a medieval castle complete with the fountain and moat. The plaque in front says, "Allie's Castle", and many people want to know what that is all about when they come to visit for the first time. They tell visitors that this was done because Alice never had the opportunity to enjoy a castle. Alice's father graciously helps Robert and Millie maintain the fountain.

In response to the medical examiner's and the county's proceedings and documents, Alice's parents wrote to their lawyers: "Responding to these documents proved to be a very time-consuming and monumental task for us, but we hope our comments assisted you in your preparation of our legal response."

Also to the lawyers: Thank you for your continued efforts on our family's behalf.

A fitting comment from the lawyers when all was finally in order again was that Carol really ought to go to law school, and they weren't kidding.

Remembrances from Grammy and Papa Anderson

When each of the Anderson's grandchildren was born, Grammy made a beautiful quilt for each of their cribs. Attached to each quilt was a poem written by Papa. The poems involved a circus parade wherein all the new baby's relatives were mentioned and ended with a happy thought for each baby's future.

My dearest Alice,

You brought us all such joy. I treasure wonderful memories of days in Florida. Your squeals of joy and laughter in our pool. You did the same when we lived in New York. The more splashing, the more waves, the more you loved it. Everyone who enjoys ice cream should learn from you, especially with lots of sprinkles. As you sit in Heaven, please know just how much we love you.

Grammy (Anderson)

Dearest Allie—

When I wrote your poem about the bears, I knew you would have "a good life". With your Mom and Dad, what else could it have been? Like Grammy, I remember how much you loved Florida. Even after a long trip, a dip in the pool was just the thing. And, of course, your smile was something we all looked forward to. You always laughed when I showed up, not even I am just sure why. But, if you didn't have a grin for me I learned when you were very young how to get one. I just beeped you. By now I'm sure, if Heaven can be improved, you have done so with your happiness and, already now, I'm sure, beeping is going on all over up there. I love you—we will have our fun times again.

Papa (Anderson)

So there you have it. This tale may not be considered to be "warm". How that could be when it deals with a medical malpractice lawsuit and a murder investigation is impossible to see. Patience and perseverance do pay off though when trying to set one's world right again. But, I guess the warmth of Alice and her family does, in the end, shine through.

Safely Home

I am home in Heaven dear ones;
Oh, so happy and so bright!
There is perfect joy and beauty
In this everlasting light.

All the pain and grief is over,
Every restless tossing passed;
I am now at peace forever,
Safely home in Heaven at last.

Author Unknown
(Dicksons)